SAGE was founded in 1965 by Sara Miller McCune to support the dissemination of usable knowledge by publishing innovative and high-quality research and teaching content. Today, we publish over 900 journals, including those of more than 400 learned societies, more than 800 new books per year, and a growing range of library products including archives, data, case studies, reports, and video. SAGE remains majority-owned by our founder, and after Sara's lifetime will become owned by a charitable trust that secures our continued independence.

Los Angeles | London | New Delhi | Singapore | Washington DC | Melbourne

Telerehabilitation
in Communication Disorders *and* Mental Health

Thank you for choosing a SAGE product!
If you have any comment, observation or feedback,
I would like to personally hear from you.

Please write to me at **contactceo@sagepub.in**

Vivek Mehra, Managing Director and CEO, SAGE India.

Bulk Sales

SAGE India offers special discounts
for purchase of books in bulk.
We also make available special imprints
and excerpts from our books on demand.

For orders and enquiries, write to us at

Marketing Department
SAGE Publications India Pvt Ltd
B1/I-1, Mohan Cooperative Industrial Area
Mathura Road, Post Bag 7
New Delhi 110044, India

E-mail us at **marketing@sagepub.in**

Subscribe to our mailing list
Write to **marketing@sagepub.in**

This book is also available as an e-book.

Telerehabilitation
in **Communication**
Disorders *and*
Mental Health

Edited by
Sanjeev Kumar Gupta

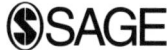

Los Angeles | London | New Delhi
Singapore | Washington DC | Melbourne

First published in 2020 by

SAGE Publications India Pvt Ltd
B1/I-1 Mohan Cooperative Industrial Area
Mathura Road, New Delhi 110 044, India
www.sagepub.in

SAGE Publications Inc
2455 Teller Road
Thousand Oaks, California 91320, USA

SAGE Publications Ltd
1 Oliver's Yard, 55 City Road
London EC1Y 1SP, United Kingdom

SAGE Publications Asia-Pacific Pte Ltd
18 Cross Street #10-10/11/12
China Square Central
Singapore 048423

Published by Vivek Mehra for SAGE Publications India Pvt Ltd and typeset in 10.5/13 pt Berkeley by AG Infographics, Delhi.

Library of Congress Cataloging-in-Publication

Names: Gupta, Sanjeev Kumar, editor.
Title: Telerehabilitation in communication disorders and mental health / Sanjeev Kumar Gupta.
Description: Thousand Oaks : SAGE Publications India Pvt Ltd, 2020. | Includes bibliographical references and index.
Identifiers: LCCN 2020008412 (print) | LCCN 2020008413 (ebook) | ISBN 9789353882778 (hardback) | ISBN 9789353882785 (epub) | ISBN 9789353882792 (ebook)
Subjects: LCSH: Communicative disorders. | Telecommunication in medicine.
Classification: LCC RC423 .T44 2020 (print) | LCC RC423 (ebook) | DDC 616.85/5–dc23
LC record available at https://lccn.loc.gov/2020008412
LC ebook record available at https://lccn.loc.gov/2020008413

ISBN: 978-93-5388-277-8 (HB)

SAGE Team: Abhijit Baroi, Syed Husain Naqvi and Abhilash Dixit

CONTENTS

LIST OF ILLUSTRATIONS

FIGURES

TABLES

LIST OF ABBREVIATIONS

%SS	Per cent syllables stuttered
AAC app	Augmentive and alternative communication app
AB	Advanced Bionics
ACT	Acceptance and commitment therapy
AIISH	All India Institute of Speech and Hearing
ANC	Active noise cancelling
AQ	Aphasia quotient
ART	Antiretroviral
ASHA	American Speech–Language–Hearing Association
AUDIT	Alcohol Use Disorders Identification Test
AUDs	Alcohol use disorders
AWS	Adults who stutter
B.ASLP	Bachelors in Audiology and Speech-Language Pathology
BBN	Broadband noise
BSPDs	Behavioural and psychological symptoms of dementia
CAI	Computer-assisted instruction
CAT for KASHI	Computerized auditory training for Kannada speaking children with hearing impairment
CBATPs	Computer-based auditory training programmes
CBT	Cognitive behavioural therapy
CET	Cue Exposure Therapy
CGs	Caregivers
CGs-PWDs	CGs of PWDs
CI	cochlear implant

CwSLD	Children with SLD
CR	Contingent reinforcement
CST	Comprehensive Stuttering Therapy
CT	Constant Therapy
CV-MAAT-K	Computerized Version of Manual for Adult Aphasia Therapy-Kannada
CWS	Children who stutter
DAF	Delayed auditory feedback
DBIS	Institute for Databases and Information Systems
DHA	Department of Health and Aging
DISHA	Digital Information Security in Healthcare Act
DPOAE	Distortion product otoacoustic emission
DSM–5®	Diagnostic and Statistical Manual of Mental Disorders
EHDI	Early Hearing Detection and Intervention
EMA	Ecological momentary assessment
EMG	Electromyographic
FDA	*Frenchay Dysarthria Assessment*
FTS	Fluency Technique Scale
GNPT	Guttmann Neuropersonal Trainer
HAP	Home auditory training programme
HD	High-definition
HL–HC	High language–high cognition
iCBT	Internet-based cognitive behavioural therapy
ICT	Information and communications technology
IP	Internet protocol
ISHA	Indian Speech and Hearing Association
ISTAR	Institute for Stuttering Treatment and Research
IT	Information technology
LL–HC	Low language–high cognition
LL–LC	Low language–low cognition
LMC	Least mean square
LPAA	Life participation approach to aphasia
MAST	Model for assessment of telemedicine applications
MLU	Mean length of utterance
NeHA	National eHealth Act
NMHS	National Mental Health Survey

NR	Non-contingent reinforcement
OPE	Oro Peripheral Examination
PHC	Primary health care centres
PRISMA	Preferred Reporting Items for Systematic Reviews and Meta-Analyses
PTA	Pure-tone audiometry
PWA	Persons with aphasia
PWDs	Persons with dementia
PWS	Person who stutters
QOL	Quality of life
RCI	Rehabilitation Council of India
RCTs	Randomized clinical trials
REELS	Receptive & Expressive Emergent Language Scale
RIDBC	Royal Institute for Deaf and Blind Children
SCRAMx	Secure Continuous Remote Alcohol Monitor
SeHA	State e-Health Act
SIG	Special interest group
SLD	Specific learning disorder
SLPs	Speech-language pathologists
SPM	Syllable per minute
SRs	Severity rating scales
SUD	Substance use disorders
SUDS	Subjective Units of Distress Scale
TBI	Traumatic brain injury
TCPD	Telecentre for Persons with Communication Disorders
TEP	Tinnitus E-Programme
TH	Telehealth
THD	Total harmonic distortions
TR	Telerehabilitation
TRI	Tinnitus Research Initiative
TXT-CBT	CBT-based text messaging intervention
TYT	Track Your Tinnitus
USCS	Urge surfing coping skills
VoIP	Voice over Internet Protocol
WAB-H	Western Aphasia Battery-Hindi

FOREWORD

Innovation distinguishes between a leader and a follower.

—Steve Jobs

Most dictionaries describe innovation as a noun. It involves the introduction of something new—an idea, a method or a device. Einstein once said, 'The true sign of intelligence is not knowledge but imagination.' Change is the crux of creativity and innovation. In the discipline of speech, language, hearing and communication disorders, for too long, traditional practices of assessment, diagnosis and intervention have ruled the roost. Traditional modes of rehabilitation suffer from inherent barriers and difficulties. *Functional barriers* are problems related to ambulating within the home or from the home to the place of service delivery. *Social barriers* can be in the form of inconvenience for the subject. There might be no caregivers to accompany them. The subject may not want to inconvenience or burden the caregivers who might be themselves busy. There can be *financial barriers*. With the rising costs of rehabilitation per session and the long duration of rehabilitation that may be needed, the time has now arrived when all this must change.

Telerehabilitation is increasingly becoming an answer to these barriers. In telerehabilitation, the therapist need not visit the patient at home or vice versa. Most of the barriers mentioned above are resolved through telerehabilitation. E-therapies are racing from the first generation (online books) to the second generation (some online interaction, learning through gaming and completing quizzes or questionnaires) to the third generation (integration with mobile phones, email and smart devices) and to the fourth generation (smart environments and mobile diagnosticians and therapists). Telerehabilitation or e-rehabilitation uses a variety of modalities via webcams, videoconferencing, phone lines, videophones and web pages with Internet applications.

The term 'telerehabilitation' has several synonyms or adjunct terms, such as teleconsultation, teleconferencing, telematics, tele-education, telemonitoring, telesupport, tele-assessment, teletherapy, telediagnosis and telecoaching. Whatever is the nomenclature, the modus operandi involves an infrastructure, forms of tele-encounter, technology access and usability, and target audience. Using e-enabled services is progress in alleviating human misery. There are no more worries regarding waiting lists or the stigma of consulting. The patient–professional contact can be tailor-made. It may be even better or more cost-effective. It helps in data compilation, storage, archiving, retrieval and corrections. Virtual reality can be made useful in treating fears and phobias for visualizing the future or reliving the past. In real time, wearable computing can help receive reality-based feedback in ameliorating conversation skills, assertiveness and emotion expression skills. Robotics is getting into place to carry out mind exercises and remind medication schedules to the forgetful elderly. For the clients, they can work at their own pace, in the privacy of their own home. Access and use of smartphones, tablets and computers is a prerequisite for telerehabilitation. Convenience, simplicity, flexibility and control, ease and entertainment are some of its apparent benefits.

Telerehabilitation is applicable in a variety of settings and clinical disciplines such as cardiology, neurology, oncology, urology, speech-language disorders, rheumatology, chronic pain, neuropsychology, mobility impairment, orthopaedics and childhood obesity, to mention a few. In spite of the glorified merits, there are many problems with new technologies. There are issues related to language and access. There is limited evidence of their effectiveness as equivalent to in-person assessment and therapy. There are ethical issues of integrating these approaches with existing practices on client privacy and monitoring. No independent bodies are in place, at least in India, to regulate these innovations. An independent policy, dedicated institution, nodal hub and funding have to be in place for the country for telerehabilitation research. Some measures, such as standards and training requirements, reimbursement policies, legislative action, professional certification and fair practices, have to be ensured. Ideally and expectedly, a combination of both processes of telerehabilitation along with traditional face-to-face consultations benefits society by reaching out to the maximum number of people in need. Such a process is likely to benefit higher numbers of people at a low cost, in quick time and with greater access, especially in Indian settings.

Against this backdrop, this book entitled *Telerehabilitation in Communication Disorders and Mental Health* is a forerunner. It treads on a path not yet entirely laid. It explores a theme that has not yet wholly taken shape. However, unperturbed and undeterred by a road not yet taken by many, Dr Sanjeev Kumar Gupta has not only authored a few critical chapters in this book but also managed to bring several specialist academicians together on a common platform as a unified team to share their insights on a contemporary theme, cutting across disciplines such as clinical psychology, audiology, speech-language pathology, special education, physiotherapy, neurology and psychiatry. The job is as challenging as the proverbial elephant being attempted to be decoded by many unsighted but eager hands. While they failed, this team has immensely succeeded, as is evidenced by this book in your hands!

Dr S. Venkatesan
Professor and Head, Department of Clinical Psychology
All India Institute of Speech and Hearing (AIISH)
Mysuru, Karnataka, India

PREFACE

Technology has become an integral part of human life. As clinicians and researchers, we have to bring innovation and new approaches in the rehabilitation services to help the masses. Therefore, the initiative to produce this book is inspired by the innovation in technology and availability of the same to the common man. The clinical services such as supervision, monitoring, consultation, assessment, diagnosis, counselling and treatment can be given to people through technology.

Research evidence suggests that early screening, identification, assessment, diagnosis and rehabilitation of persons with communication disorders and mental health issues can help affected people to improve the quality of life and lessen the economic and social burden on the caregiver. The caregiver is the backbone for the treatment. Therefore, the training of the parent or caregiver in technology usage is the need of the hour for the sustainable rehabilitation of people. A conducive environment for people is effective not only for physical well-being but also for mental health. A multidisciplinary team can be helpful to deal with most of the aspects of communication disorders and mental health issues.

This book offers a wide range of useful and interesting topics in the area of telerehabilitation in communication disorders and mental health such as telepractice in speech-language pathology, tele-audiology in India, telerehabilitation in stuttering, tele-special education, telerehabilitation in aphasia, dementia, specific learning disabilities and substance use disorders, to name a few. It can be used as a stepping stone for further research and clinical practice in the field of telerehabilitation.

In conclusion, as a comprehensive collection of recent research findings, this book provides researchers, practitioners, academicians, health care professionals and policymakers a good understanding of applications, issues and challenges of telerehabilitation about communication disorders and mental health.

ACKNOWLEDGEMENTS

The process of producing a new book is always a challenging but rewarding academic work and requires mutual support from the contributors, reviewers and stakeholders for the quality of the content and timely completion of the book.

First and foremost, I would like to thank all the contributors for their research contributions and scientific knowledge, which they have meticulously put into the chapters. I thank and acknowledge the active involvement of the reviewers for the improvement of the quality, coherence and content of the chapters.

I am also thankful to Dr M. Pushpavathi, Director, AIISH, Mysuru, and Dr S. Venkatesan, Head of the Department of Clinical Psychology, AIISH, for providing me with the needful support while working on the book.

Finally, I sincerely thank the SAGE team for their guidance and support through the editing and publication of the book.

Telerehabilitation
Emerging Opportunities and Challenges

Sanjeev Kumar Gupta

INTRODUCTION

According to the Census of India, there are 26.81 million people with disabilities who constitute 2.21 per cent of the total population. Out of the total persons with disabilities, 1.5 million (5.61%) have mental retardation/intellectual disability and 1.99 million have speech-related disability (Office of the Registrar General & Census Commissioner, India 2013). However, a new World Bank report on disability in India shows increasing evidence of people with disabilities which comprise between 5 and 8 per cent of the Indian population (O'Keefe 2007). It is also estimated that 15 per cent of the world's population has some form of disability (World Health Organization 2011). The application of TR offers effective solutions to this challenge.

Recent developments and innovations in information and communication technology (ICT) are transforming the landscape of TR service delivery all over the world. TR is one of the rapidly growing methods of providing rehabilitation services over telecommunication networks and the Internet. Many terms are commonly and interchangeably used in the health care set-up such as e-health, m-health, telepractice, telehealth, telemodel, teleconsultation, telehomecare and telemonitoring to name a few (Larson et al. 2014). All of the above-given terms or modalities can be a subcategory of TR and would come under the broader category of telemedicine (Khanna et al. 2018). Telemedicine is defined as 'transfer or exchange of medical and health care information using ICT' (Brennan, Mawson and Brownsell 2009).

The term 'telerehabilitation' is made up of two words tele and rehabilitation. The prefix *tele* is a Greek word for distant or remote

(Darkins and Cary 2000). It is used to explain the transfer of information over a distance, like a telephone (Houston 2013). The word 'rehabilitation' comes from the Latin word *rehabilitationem* meaning 'restoration'. So, the word 'telerehabilitation' refers to restoring or regaining or improving the lost or diminished functions through the delivery of rehabilitation services over the Internet or telecommunication networks. TR is also defined as 'delivery of intervention services to the person at their location using ICT' (Brennan, Mawson and Brownsell 2009).

TR refers to the rehabilitation and habilitation services through Internet and may include health education, counselling, guidance, consultations, supervision, monitoring, clinical assessments, interventions and follow-ups. TR services are used in the areas of neuropsychology, speech-language pathology, occupational therapy, audiology, neurology, psychotherapy, psychiatry and physical therapy. The most commonly used modalities for TR are smartphones, webcams and videoconferencing. Research evidence supports the fact that rehabilitation services delivered in a patient's natural environment like home are more effective than the same treatment delivered in a hospital or clinic (McCue et al. 2010). TR may be an important therapeutic module to reduce the cost of the treatment which in turn may reduce the caregiver's economic burden. TR can be a viable option to improve community-based rehabilitation systems, particularly in the developing countries where rehabilitation services are expensive and not available at the community level (Kairy et al. 2009). The use of TR may revolutionize health care set-up. However, there is an urgent need for future studies of good-quality TR, analysing its cost-benefits and cost-effectiveness for the benefit of the society at large (Shenoy and Shenoy 2018).

Health professionals can identify the need to reach the unreached in India by using a 'telerehabilitation model' for the intervention of persons with communication disorders (Rangaswamy and Rao 2018) and mental health issues. This chapter discusses the utility and importance of TR in speech-language pathology and audiology, in mental health and in South Asia, and the guidelines, challenges, advantages and barriers in providing TR services.

TELEREHABILITATION IN SPEECH-LANGUAGE PATHOLOGY AND AUDIOLOGY

The use and importance of telepractice in the discipline of speech-language pathology was identified more than two decades ago. However, the recent advancement in the field of ICT has completely changed the scope and utility of telepractice of speech-language pathology in health professions (Theodoros 2011). Despite the challenges in the discipline of speech-language pathology and audiology, clinical service delivery through telemodel is positively embraced in India (Rangaswamy and Rao 2018).

Telemedicine or use of interactive videoconferencing is reported to be effective in the assessment and successful intervention of stuttering in children and adolescents (Sicotte et al. 2003). Computer-based language therapy has shown good results in aphasia (Cherney et al. 2008). The Hindi version of Constant Therapy (CT), an iPad software platform on a set of 20 tasks spread across a span of 3–5 sessions, is used in persons with aphasia. The study highlighted the importance of knowing the benefits of aphasia therapy in rehabilitation, family support and assistance by the therapist to maintain good compliance to therapy (Kasturi and Goswami 2019). Numerous innovations in the tele speech-language pathology (Theodoros 2011) and audiology are yet to be realized.

TELEREHABILITATION IN MENTAL HEALTH

Telepsychology or Telemental Health

Telepsychology is defined as 'mental health care services through information communication technologies with or without traditional face-to-face methods (American Psychological Association, n.d.).' In other words, telepsychology refers to the use of technology-assisted devices to provide mental health services (Rees and Haythornthwaite 2011). Telepsychology and telepsychiatry applications are accepted by the clients and professionals (Cullum et al. 2014).

Research evidence supports the fact that telepsychology is effective in the treatment of public speaking fear (Botella et al. 2007) and posttraumatic stress disorder (Bolton and Dorstyn 2015). Tata Institute of Social Sciences, Mumbai, has set up iCALL—a psychosocial helpline to address the mental health needs of the people in India. iCALL offers individual counselling by telephone and email modalities (Sriram, Joshi and Sharma 2016). Depression related free mobile apps for Indian users were reviewed and studied to help people with depression. These apps can be downloaded on an Android phone (Kumar and Mehrotra 2017).

Teleneuropsychology

Cognitive impairment occurs in multiple sclerosis (Chiaravalloti and DeLuca 2008), traumatic brain injury (Arciniegas, Held and Wagner 2002; Soeda et al. 2005), schizophrenia (Elvevag and Goldberg 2000; Schaefer et al. 2013) and many other clinical conditions. Traditional approaches for cognitive remediation are time-consuming, expensive and difficult to uniformly implement (Rosti Otajärvi and Hämäläinen 2014) and evaluate, but some trials benefit the client. TR can optimize the sequencing of intervention, intensity, timing and lead to the greatest functional result for the patient (Winters and Winters 2004).

Computer-based cognitive remediation programme accessed from home can be effective in improving cognitive functions in persons with multiple sclerosis (Charvet et al. 2017). Cognitive rehabilitation is commonly used in the case of acquired brain injury to remediate cognitive deficits. Solana et al. (2015) described Guttmann Neuropersonal Trainer (GNPT). It allows neuropsychologists to customize treatment plans, provide information to further development of the practice guidelines and to configure and schedule training sessions. The GNPT provides remote access and continuous monitoring of the client's performance. Video teleconference-based neuropsychological assessment is a reliable and valid alternative to conventional face-to-face assessment using selected measures (Cullum et al. 2014). Research studies suggest that TR services are effective, feasible and less resource-intensive in delivering quality health care in India (Khanna et al. 2018).

Telepsychotherapy

Telepsychotherapy is defined as conducting psychotherapy sessions through advanced technology and supporting real-time interactivity (Kaplan 1997). Studies supported the notion that therapeutic alliance can be developed in psychotherapy through videoconferencing (Simpson and Reid 2014).

Smartphones can be used as an extension of psychotherapy to help patients (Chan et al. 2014). The two retrospective studies presenting computer-based psychological intervention for comorbid depression and substance use disorder (Kay-Lambkin et al. 2009), and Internet-based CBT for panic disorder and agoraphobia (Kiropoulos et al. 2008) have shown that the outcome was found to be comparable to that of face to face methods.

Eshwarage and Gunesekara (2017) developed a Web-based expert system which will provide personalized psychotherapeutic counselling for the Sri Lankan community. The system presents a set of standards and psychologically-approved questions to the clients before they receive the counselling service. By using Prolog Logical Programming Language, the answers provided by the client are analysed and then the system predicts the area of the problem of that particular client. The system, then, directs the client to the relevant counsellor who has specialized in that relevant area. Finally, the client could use a preferred method of communication, facilitated by the system, to communicate with the counsellor.

Telepsychiatry

Parents were highly satisfied with the health care given to their children by using interactive videos, thus illustrating evidence that telepsychiatry is an effective tool to increase access to underserved youth and the spectrum of their needs (Myers, Valentine and Melzer 2008).

Yellowlees and Chan (2015) explained that in a country like India where health providers are scarce, mobile applications are easily available and can connect patients with other patients, families, caregivers and supporters through social media. With multiple educational and monitoring programmes designed to prevent psychiatric disorders, these apps can improve medication adherence and provide social support and therapy.

Telerehabilitation for Geriatric Problems

Inaccessibility, dependency on caregivers and healthcare costs are the challenges faced by the geriatric population in low and middle-income countries. Due to these factors, elders are unwilling to engage in rehabilitation and preventive health programmes. Therefore there is a need to identify alternative methods of health promotion services and TR is one such method (Narekuli, Raja and Pandve 2019).

Narekuli, Raja and Pandve (2019) studied to identify the barriers to videoconferencing, which is an easy method of TR delivery. This study was a cross-sectional survey using interview and observation methods. The study suggests that training on how to use the technology is essential. Establishment of prerequisites before the actual delivery of TR may potentially increase acceptability and hence sustainability. TR is in practice for the care of older persons. There is evidence that TR can foster the resumption of activities of daily living of older persons and therefore, can improve their lifestyle and social integration (Gregory, Alexander and Satinsky 2011).

TELEREHABILITATION IN SOUTH ASIA

TR is presently used in India (Kasturi and Goswami 2019; Rangaswamy and Rao 2018), Bangladesh (Hasan, Khan and Uddin 2012), Pakistan (Khan et al. 2017) and Sri Lanka (Eshwarage and Gunesekara 2017).

In India, there is a great disparity in quality and access to healthcare between urban and rural areas (Vijitha 2018). Therefore, TR can be one of the methods to improve the health status of the Indian population. The telecentre for persons with communication disorders (TCPD) is one of the departments at All India Institute of Speech and Hearing

(AIISH), Mysuru, which delivers teleservices such as consultation, assessment, counselling and rehabilitation services via telepractice modality, for the persons with communication disorders. The Tata Institute of Social Sciences, Mumbai, runs iCALL— a psychosocial helpline through telephone and email for the persons with mental health issues (Sriram, Joshi and Sharma 2016).

Very few studies are being reported in India on TR (Rao, Iyer and Anap 2012). However, the interest is growing exponentially in this area. TCPD at AIISH is also actively engaged in conducting the research in the area of tele speech-language pathology and audiology (Rangaswamy and Rao 2018). Ayanikalath, Pillay and Jayaram (2018) tried to identify various factors by using the semi-structured interviews of TR personnel to study the factors that influence the effectiveness of TR.

In Bangladesh, Hasan, Khan and Uddin (2012) designed and implemented a TR programme on hand skill development for the persons with disabilities. They have used the user-centred design model to develop the programme.

In Pakistan, the field of rehabilitation sciences is under development, but still, have great career opportunities and scope (Babur 2017). The use of TR needs more consideration in Pakistan, especially in rural areas. TR is also poorly integrated with the country's acute care system (Khan et al. 2017).

In Sri Lanka, Eshwarage and Gunesekara (2017) examined the development of a web-based expert system which provides personalized psychotherapeutic counselling for the Sri Lankan community. Durrani and Khoja (2009) conducted a systematic review of the literature on telehealth in Asia and reported that the number of published research articles on telehealth increased in Asia.

GUIDELINES FOR TELEREHABILITATION PRACTICE

AIISH, Mysuru published guidelines for service delivery through telepractice modality. These guidelines are strictly followed at the TCPD. Guidelines and frameworks are also needed to evaluate apps and softwares (Chan et al. 2015).

The members of the American Telemedicine Association, with input from other professionals in the field and strategic stakeholders, developed the guidelines for TR to assist practitioners in providing safe and effective services (Brennan et al. 2010). The guidelines represent clinical, administrative, ethical and technical principles that should be considered in the course of providing TR services, for further reading refer to Brennan et al. (2010).

CHALLENGES IN TELEREHABILITATION

Following are the challenges in TR:

- Lack of TR protocols in India
- Patients' acceptance
- Reimbursement and insurance
- Licensure
- Medico-legal issues
- Costs of implementation
- Security and privacy issues
- Professional acceptance
- Technical challenges
- Concerns about client confidentiality (Rangaswamy and Rao 2018)

ADVANTAGE OF TELEREHABILITATION

- Facilitating the cost-effective availability of TR services
- Reaching out TR services in remote and rural locations with flexible scheduling where health professionals are not available
- Taking TR services to persons with mobility problems who cannot contact health professionals
- Providing individualized assessment and intervention services according to the learning style and pace of the person via TR
- Mobile applications are portable and easily connect health care providers with the client (Yellowlees and Chan 2015)
- Access therapy in a native language such as the Hindi version of CT (Kasturi and Goswami 2019)

BARRIERS TO TELEREHABILITATION

- Scarce availability of necessary technological facilities in semi-urban and rural locales
- Lack of computer literacy and technical ignorance among service receivers and caregivers
- High cost involved in availing necessary technological devices and arranging teleservices
- Lack of awareness about teleservices among the general public, as well as the stakeholders

CONCLUSION

The trained and experienced mental health and rehabilitation professionals are scanty in India. Therefore, the use of TR activities in delivering clinical services would be a feasible option to cater the needs of the larger number of people seeking rehabilitation services in the areas of speech and language disorders, neuropsychological rehabilitation, psychotherapy and community-based rehabilitation. It is cost-effective, fast, time-saving and can also be integrated with traditional face to face treatment. However, further research work is warranted to promote, evaluate and analyse the efficacy and effectiveness of TR.

REFERENCES

American Psychological Association. n.d. 'What are Telehealth and Telepsychology?' Available at: https://www.apa.org/pi/disability/resources/publications/telepsychology (accessed on 18 December 2019).

Arciniegas, David B., Kerri Held, and Peter Wagner. 2002. 'Cognitive Impairment Following Traumatic Brain Injury.' *Current Treatment Options in Neurology* 4 (1): 43–57. doi: 10.1007/s11940-002-0004-6

Ayanikalath, Sona, Mershen Pillay, and M. Jayaram. 2018. 'Is India Ready for Telerehabilitation?' Available at: http://www.indianjournals.com/ijor.asp x?target=ijor:ijphrd&volume=9&issue=11&article=035 (accessed on 18 December 2019).

Babur, Muhammad Naveed. 2017. 'Evolution, Innovation & Transformation Of Rehabilitation Sciences in Pakistan.' Available at: http://ijrs.org/ojs/index.php/ IJRS/article/view/94 (accessed on 18 December 2019).

Bolton, A. J., and D. S. Dorstyn. 2015. 'Telepsychology for Posttraumatic Stress Disorder: A Systematic Review.' Available at: https://journals.sagepub.com/doi/abs/10.1177/1357633X15571996 (accessed on 18 December 2019).

Botella, Cristina, Veronica Guillen, Rosa M. Banos, Azucena García-Palacios, Maria J. Gallego, and Mariano Alcanizc. 2007. 'Telepsychology and Self-help: The Treatment of Fear of Public Speaking.' Available at: https://www.sciencedirect.com/science/article/abs/pii/S107772290600126X (accessed on 18 December 2019).

Brennan, David, Lyn Tindall, Deborah Theodoros, Janet Brown, Michael Campbell, Diana Christiana, David Smith, Jana Cason and Alan Lee. 2010. 'A Blueprint for Telerehabilitation Guidelines.' Available at: https://www.ncbi.nlm.nih.gov/pmc/articles/PMC4296793/ (accessed on 18 December 2019).

Brennan, David, Sue Mawson, and Simon Brownsell. 2009. 'Telerehabilitation: Enabling the Remote Delivery of Healthcare, Rehabilitation, and Self Management.' *Studies in Health Technology and Informatics* 145: 231–248.

Chan, Steven Richard, John Torous, Ladson Hinton, and Peter Yellowlees. 2014. 'Mobile Tele-Mental Health: Increasing Applications and a Move to Hybrid Models of Care.' *Healthcare* 2 (2): 220–233. doi: 10.3390/healthcare2020220

Chan, Steven Richard, John Torous, Ladson Hinton, and Peter Yellowlees. 2015. 'Towards a Framework for Evaluating Mobile Mental Health Apps.' *Telemedicine and e-Health* 21 (12): 1038–1041. Available at: https://doi.org/10.1089/tmj.2015.0002 (accessed on 18 December 2019).

Charvet, Leigh E., Jie Yang, Michael T. Shaw, Kathleen Sherman, Lamia Haider, Jianjin Xu, and Lauren B. Krupp. 2017. 'Cognitive Function in Multiple Sclerosis Improves with Telerehabilitation: Results from a Randomized Controlled Trial.' *PLoS ONE* 12 (5): e0177177. doi: 10.1371/journal.pone.0177177

Cherney, Leora R., Anita S. Halper, Audrey L. Holland, and Ron Cole. 2008. 'Computerized Script Training for Aphasia: Preliminary Results.' Available at: https://pubs.asha.org/doi/10.1044/1058-0360(2008/003) (accessed on 18 December 2019).

Chiaravalloti, Nancy D., and John DeLuca. 2008. 'Cognitive Impairment in Multiple Sclerosis.' *The Lancet Neurology* 7 (12): 1139–1151. doi: 10.1016/S1474-4422(08)70259-X

Cullum, C. Munro, L. S. Hynan, M. Grosch, and M. Parikh. 2014. 'Teleneuropsychology: Evidence for Video Teleconference-based Neuropsychological Assessment.' doi: 10.1017/S1355617714000873

Darkins, Adam William, and Margaret Ann Cary. 2000. *Telemedicine and Telehealth: Principles, Policies, Performances and Pitfalls.* London: Free Association Books.

Durrani, Hammad, and Shariq Khoja. 2009. 'A Systematic Review of the Use of Telehealth in Asian Countries.' Available at: https://journals.sagepub.com/doi/abs/10.1258/jtt.2009.080605 (accessed on 18 December 2019).

Elvevag, Brita, and Terry E. Goldberg. 2000. 'Cognitive Impairment in Schizophrenia is the Core of the Disorder.' *Critical Reviews in Neurobiology* 14 (1). doi: 10.1615/CritRevNeurobiol.v14.i1.10

Eshwarage, Sahani, and A. Gunesekara. 2017. 'Web-Based Expert System for Personalized Psychotherapeutic Counselling.' Available at: http://ir.kdu.ac.lk/handle/345/1680 (accessed on 18 December 2019).

Gregory, Patricia, Joshua Alexander, and Jennifer Satinsky. 2011. 'Clinical Telerehabilitation: Applications for Physiatrists.' Available at: https://www.sciencedirect.com/science/article/abs/pii/S1934148211001729 (accessed on 18 December 2019).

Hasan, Mahmud, Jahidul I. Khan, and Md. Sami Uddin. 2012. 'Designing and Implementing Telerehabilitation on Hand Skill Development for the Disabled People in Bangladesh.' Available at: http://ijse.org.eg/papers/designing-and-implementing-telerehabilitation-on-hand-skill-development-for-the-disabled-people-in-bangladesh/ (accessed on 12 January 2019).

Houston, K. Todd. 2013. *Telepractice in Speech-Language Pathology.* San Diego, California: Plural Publishing, Inc.

Kairy, Dahlia, Pascale Lehoux, Claude Vincent, and Martha Visintin. 2009. 'A Systematic Review of Clinical Outcomes, Clinical Process, Healthcare Utilization and Costs Associated with Telerehabilitation.' *Disability and Rehabilitation* 31 (6): 427–447. doi: 10.1080/09638280802062553

Kaplan, E. H. 1997, Summer. 'Telepsychotherapy. Psychotherapy by Telephone, Videotelephone, and Computer Videoconferencing.' Available at: https://www.ncbi.nlm.nih.gov/pmc/articles/PMC3330458/ (accessed on 18 December 2019).

Kasturi, Vimala J., and S. P. Goswami. 2019. 'Task Compliance to App-Based Rehabilitation in Persons with Aphasia in India.' *International Journal of Mind, Brain & Cognition* 10 (1–2): 96–108.

Kay-Lambkin, Frances J., Amanda L. Baker, Terry J. Lewin, and Vaughan J. Carr. 2009. 'Computer-based Psychological Treatment for Comorbid Depression and Problematic Alcohol and/or Cannabis Use: A Randomized Controlled Trial of Clinical Efficacy.' Available at: https://onlinelibrary.wiley.com/doi/abs/10.1111/j.1360-0443.2008.02444.x (accessed on 18 December 2019).

Khan F., Amatya B., Sayed T. M., Butt A. W., Jamil K., Iqbal W., Elmalik A., Rathore F. A., and Abbott G. 2017. 'World Health Organization Global Disability Action Plan 2014–2021: Challenges and Perspective for Physical Medicine and Rehabilitation in Pakistan.' *Ingenta Connect.* Available at: https://www.ingentaconnect.com/contentone/mjl/sreh/2017/00000049/00000001/art00003 (accessed on 18 December 2019).

Khanna, M., G. S. Gowda, V. I. Bagevadi, A. Gupta, K. Kulkarni, R. P. S. Shyam, and V. Basavaraju. 2018. 'Feasibility and Utility of Tele-Neurorehabilitation Service in India: Experience from a Quaternary Center.' Available at: https://www.ncbi.nlm.nih.gov/pmc/articles/PMC6126315/ (accessed on 18 December 2019).

Kiropoulos, PanelLitza A., Britt Klein, David W. Austin, Kathryn Gilson, Ciaran Pier, Joanna Mitchell, and Lisa Ciechomski. 2008. 'Is Internet-Based CBT for Panic Disorder and Agoraphobia as Effective as Face-to-Face CBT?' Available at: https://www.sciencedirect.com/science/article/abs/pii/S0887618508000170 (accessed on 18 December 2019).

Kumar, Satish, and Seema Mehrotra. 2017. 'Free Mobile Apps on Depression for Indian Users: A Brief Overview and Critique.' Available at: https://www.sciencedirect.com/science/article/abs/pii/S1876201816306013 (accessed on 18 December 2019).

Larson, Eric B., Maia Feigon, Pablo Gagliardo, and Assaf Y. Dvorkin. 2014. 'Virtual Reality and Cognitive Rehabilitation: A Review of Current Outcome Research—IOS Press.' Available at: https://content.iospress.com/articles/neurorehabilitation/nre1078 (accessed on 18 December 2019).

McCue, Michael, Andrea Fairman, Michael Pramuka, and PlumX Metrics. 2010. 'Enhancing Quality of Life through Telerehabilitation.' *Physical Medicine and Rehabilitation Clinics of North America* 21 (1): 195–205. Available at: https://www.sciencedirect.com/science/article/abs/pii/S104796510900059X?via%3Dihub (accessed on 18 December 2019).

Myers, Kathleen M., Jeanette M. Valentine, and Sanford M. Melzer. 2008. 'Child and Adolescent Telepsychiatry: Utilization And Satisfaction.' Available at: https://www.liebertpub.com/doi/abs/10.1089/tmj.2007.0035 (accessed on 18 December 2019).

Narekuli, Anushree, Kavitha Raja, and Harshal Tukaram Pandve. 2019. 'Telerehabilitation in India: Points to Ponder.' *Indian Journal of Physiotherapy and Occupational Therapy* 13 (3): 18–21 Available at: https://www.indian-journals.com/ijor.aspx?target=ijor:ijpot&volume=13&issue=3&article=004 (accessed on 18 December 2019).

Office of the Registrar General & Census Commissioner, India. 2013. *2011 Census Data*. Available at: http://www.censusindia.gov.in/2011-Common/CensusData2011.html (accessed on 18 December 2019).

O'Keefe, P. 2007. 'People with Disabilities in India: From Commitments to Outcomes.' Available at: https://scholar.google.com/scholar?hl=en&as_sdt=0%2C5&q=People+with+disabilities+in+India%3A+from+commitments+to+outcomes&btnG = (accessed on 18 December 2019).

Rangaswamy, Yashaswini, and Prema K. S. Rao. 2018. 'Tele Speech-Language Pathology and Audiology in India—a Short Report.' *Journal of the International Society for Telemedicine and EHealth* 6 (November): e19 (1–8).

Rao, Keerthi, Chandra Iyer, and Deepak Anap. 2012. 'Can Telerehabilitation Add a New Dimension in the Treatment of Osteoarthritis Knee?' Available at: https://www.omicsonline.org/peer-reviewed/can-telerehabilitation-add-a-new-dimension-in-the-treatment-of-osteoarthritis-kneep-9484.html (accessed on 18 December 2019).

Rees, Clare S., and Sarah Haythornthwaite. 2011. 'Telepsychology and Videoconferencing: Issues, Opportunities and Guidelines for Psychologists.'

Australian Psychologist 39 (3): 212–219. Available at: https://aps.onlinelibrary.wiley.com/doi/abs/10.1080/00050060412331295108 (accessed on 18 December 2019).

Rosti Otajärvi, Eija M., and Päivi I. Hämäläinen. 2014. 'Neuropsychological Rehabilitation for Multiple Sclerosis.' *Cochrane Database of Systematic Reviews*, no. 2. doi: 10.1002/14651858.CD009131.pub3

Schaefer, Jonathan, Evan Giangrande, Daniel R. Weinberger, and Dwight Dickinson. 2013. 'The Global Cognitive Impairment in Schizophrenia: Consistent over Decades and around the World.' *Schizophrenia Research*, DSM–5, 150 (1): 42–50. doi: 10.1016/j.schres.2013.07.009

Shenoy, Manisha Pramod, and Pramod Divakara Shenoy. 2018. 'Identifying the Challenges and Cost-Effectiveness of Telerehabilitation: A Narrative Review.' 2018. Available at: https://www.researchgate.net/publication/329752089_Identifying_the_challenges_and_cost-effectiveness_of_telerehabilitation_A_narrative_review (accessed on 18 December 2019).

Sicotte, Claude, Pascale Lehoux, Julie Fortier-Blanc, and Yves Leblanc. 2003. 'Feasibility and Outcome Evaluation of a Telemedicine Application in Speech–Language Pathology.' Available at: https://journals.sagepub.com/doi/abs/10.1258/135763303769211256 (accessed on 18 December 2019).

Simpson, Susan G., and Corinne L. Reid. 2014. 'Therapeutic Alliance in Videoconferencing Psychotherapy: A Review.' Available at: https://onlinelibrary.wiley.com/doi/abs/10.1111/ajr.12149 (accessed on 18 December 2019).

Soeda, Akio, Toshihiko Nakashima, Ayumi Okumura, Kazuo Kuwata, Jun Shinoda, and Toru Iwama. 2005. 'Cognitive Impairment after Traumatic Brain Injury: A Functional Magnetic Resonance Imaging Study Using the Stroop Task.' *Neuroradiology* 47 (7): 501–506. doi: 10.1007/s00234-005-1372-x

Solana, J., C. Cáceres, A. García-Molina, E. Opisso, T. Roig, J. M. Tormos, and E. J. Gómez. 2015. 'Improving Brain Injury Cognitive Rehabilitation by Personalized Telerehabilitation Services: Guttmann Neuropersonal Trainer.' *IEEE Journal of Biomedical and Health Informatics* 19 (1): 124–131. doi: 10.1109/JBHI.2014.2354537

Sriram, Sujata, Aparna Joshi, and Paras Sharma. 2016. 'Telephone Counselling in India: Lessons from iCALL.' Available at: https://link.springer.com/chapter/10.1007/978-981-10-0584-8_11 (accessed on 18 December 2019).

Theodoros, Deborah. 2011. 'Telepractice in Speech-Language Pathology: The Evidence, the Challenges, and the Future.' Available at: https://lshss.pubs.asha.org/doi/full/10.1044/tele1.1.10 (accessed on 18 December 2019).

Vijitha, Burra. 2018. 'Impact of E-Health Technology in India.' SSRN Scholarly Paper ID 3197079. Rochester, NY: Social Science Research Network. Available at: https://papers.ssrn.com/abstract=3197079 (accessed on 18 December 2019).

Winters, Jack M., and Jill M. Winters. 2004. 'A Telehomecare Model for Optimizing Rehabilitation Outcomes.' Available at: https://www.liebertpub.com/doi/abs/10.1089/tmj.2004.10.200 (accessed on 18 December 2019).

World Health Organization. 2011. 'World Report on Disability.' Available at: https://www.who.int/disabilities/world_report/2011/report/en/ (accessed on 18 December 2019).

Yellowlees, Peter, and Steven Chan. 2015. 'Mobile Mental Health Care—an Opportunity for India.' *The Indian Journal of Medical Research* 142 (4): 359–361. Available at: http://www.ijmr.org.in/article.asp?issn=09715916;year=2015;volume=142;issue=4;spage=359;epage=361;aulast=Yellowlees (accessed on 18 December 2019).

Telerehabilitation in Communication Disorders

1

Telepractice in Speech-Language Pathology in India

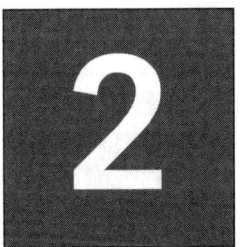

*Attuluri Navya, G. Swetha,
Pratiksha Gupta and
Pebbili Gopikishore*

INTRODUCTION

Technological advancements have made life easier and more comfortable. Especially the various forms of 'tele' communications have reached greater heights with the advent of the audio and video transmissions in real-time. The Greek word *tele* means remote or distant (Darkins and Cary 2000) and this is used to transfer information over a distance through telegraph, telephone and television. According to American Speech and Hearing Association (ASHA 2004), telepractice in the field of speech-language pathology is to provide professional services at a distance mode by connecting the clinician with the client as shown in Figure 2.1. In addition to that, clinicians also can share and discuss the evaluation reports and can plan treatment strategies. In the 1990s, with the advent of the Internet, the federal departments, military, profit and non-profit organizations and universities started studying and supporting telepractice models for medical services. The rapid use of broadband Internet connections enabled connected communication and information sharing across the countries of the world.

India is one of the fastest developing countries of the world with a total population of 1.34 billion (India Census data 2011). Recent census results suggest that 2.13 per cent (India Census Data 2011) and 1.8 per cent (NSSO GOI 2002) of the Indian population is affected with a disability. Approximately 4 per cent of the population have communication disorders (Rao and Yashaswini 2019, 67). To cater to the needs of a huge population with disability, the number

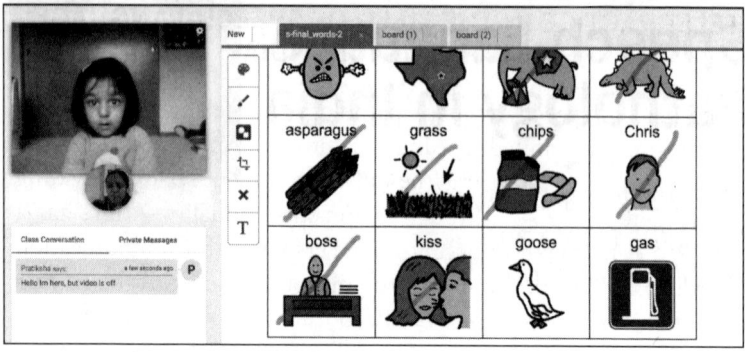

Figure 2.1 *A Client Receiving Speech Therapy through Telepractice Model*

of rehabilitation professionals, especially speech-language pathologists (SLPs) are only 1:32,000 (Rao and Yashaswini 2019, 67). The
disproportion could be due to the brain drain of the speech-language
pathologists and audiologists. The results of a survey on the professionals graduated from a premier institute in India reported nearly 81
per cent of brain drain (Savithri and Jayaram 2003).

In this scenario, the technological advancements in telecommunications in India are well known with 931.95 million telephone
subscribers (Telecom Regulatory Authority of India 2014). The afford-
ability of the Internet services encourages the professionals and the
clients to use various free and paid platforms for videoconferencing
such as Skype, Google Hangouts, Zoom, LINE, Tango, IMO, Adobe
Connect Pro, CISCO Webex and SCOPIA. Most of these applications
can be used on mobiles, tablets, desktops and laptops for video calling. Some of these software packages do have provisions for sharing
PowerPoints, documents, group chatting and a whiteboard to scribble
and for recording live sessions.

In 2015, the Indian government took initiative to encourage
eHealth and telemedicine practices through Digital India programme
in coordination with National Informatics Centre. Through this programme, telemedicine services are provided via the eHospital website:
https://ehospital.nic.in/ehospitalsso/. This has opened an avenue to
receive online medical services from 321 hospitals and more than
76,903,031 patients availed medical services since 2015.

TELEPRACTICE IN THE FIELD OF SPEECH-LANGUAGE PATHOLOGY IN INDIA

In the field of speech-language pathology, the telepractice services in India are very limited. All India Institute of Speech and Hearing (AIISH) located in Mysuru is the only government set-up providing speech therapy services through telepractice modality. AIISH has a dedicated department (Telecentre for Persons with Communication Disorders-TCPD) focusing on providing telepractice through two modalities. The clients who can afford to have personalized systems at home can avail the services directly, others with lack of resources can avail the services through nearby hospitals which are in coordination with the TCPD at AIISH. They provide evaluations, rehabilitation and educational guidance through telepractice modality. In addition to these, there is a dedicated helpline and a website to serve clients with Parkinson's disease.

Other private educational institutions providing telepractice are Sri Ramachandra Medical College (SRMC), Chennai and Bhartiya Vidyapeeth University, Pune. 1SpecialPlace (https://1specialplace.com) is one of the largest private organizations doing multidisciplinary clinical work in telepractice in India. They provide speech-language therapy, occupational therapy, special education and psychology services all under one umbrella. They have conducted more than 3,000 online sessions by the end of the year 2018 and have seen patients from 50 cities in the country. Their screening app Speech Doctor, which can identify speech and language difficulties, offers simple app-based diagnostics and self-help remedies backed by reliable data. Speech Doctor is an app that assists parents and speech therapists alike in the identification of speech-related disorders in kids at an early stage. Through the app, a parent or a doctor can get a fair idea of whether the child under his/her care needs special speech and language enrichment. The app tests both receptive and expressive language skills in children. It is a freely downloadable app on the App store.

A survey questionnaire related to telepractice in speech-language pathology and audiology was circulated to the members of Indian Speech and Hearing Association (ISHA) by Mohan, Anjum and Rao (2017). The results indicated that out of 2,800 registered members, only 205 SLPs and audiologists responded and it was noticed that only 12.19 per cent (25 out of 205) were engaged in telepractice. Among these 25 professionals, only 12 were rendering speech-language pathology services, three were providing audiological services and 10 were involved in both speech-language pathology and audiological services. Another interesting fact noticed was that out of these 25 professionals, 14 were serving through telepractice within India, remaining 11 were serving from other countries. The majority of the patients enrolled for services through telepractice mode were with speech sound disorders followed by learning disabilities and childhood language disorders. On the contrary, less number of children with motor speech disorders and auditory processing disorders were enrolled for telepractice. This could also be because the former disorders are more prevalent than latter.

A patient satisfaction survey was conducted in India by 1SpecialPlace (2018) for 40 patients availing speech therapy services through telepractice model and a couple of patients' testimonials are in Appendix B. In a recent survey the patients were asked the following questions and were requested to rate the answers on a scale of 1–5, where, 1 corresponded to poor and 5 meant excellent.

1. Technical quality of sessions
2. Rate your therapist
3. Involvement of the parent/caregiver
4. Progress after therapy
5. Interest in the sessions
6. Overall rating

All clients reported satisfactory quality of sessions and good progress after the therapy sessions. Technical quality was the only question which yielded 3, 4 and 5 ratings. This can be attributed to the fluctuating Internet services at some patients' end during the course of therapy sessions. While on the other hand, all other questions were rated 4 or 5. Most of the clients gave a score of 5 to their therapist and expressed that the patient was engaged very well in the sessions. Involvement of caregiver was scored 4 or 5 by all the clients.

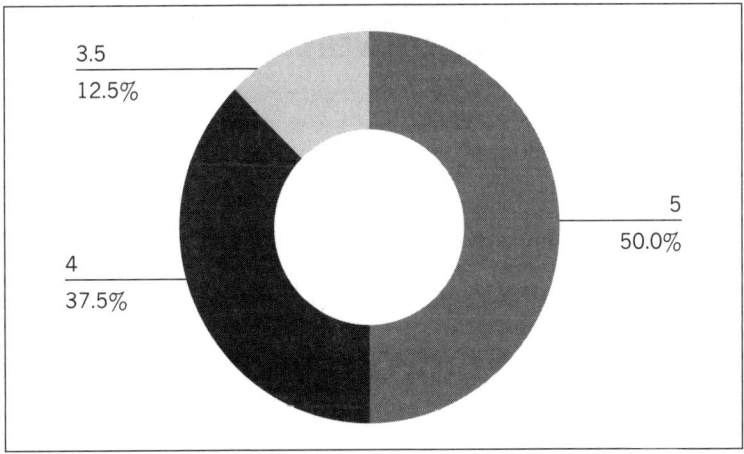

Figure 2.2 *Overall Rating for the Speech Therapy Received through Telepractice Model by the Clients*

The overall ratings of half of the clients (50%) corresponded to excellent and 37.5 per cent of clients rated 4 points out of 5 whereas only 12.5 per cent of clients rated 3.5 as shown in Figure 2.2.

INDIAN POLICIES FOR TELEPRACTICE

- In 2017, AIISH published policies for telepractice. These guidelines are being followed at the TCPD. The policy framework is divided into following heads; administrative, clinical, technical and ethical.
- The Ministry of Health and Family Welfare launched the Digital Information Security in Healthcare Act (DISHA) which enables digital sharing of personal health records between hospitals and clinics, and vice versa. It will help in maintaining the confidentiality, privacy and security of electronic health data.
- The National eHealth Act (NeHA) was set up in 2015 as a promotional, regulatory and standards-setting organization in the healthcare sector.
- The State eHealth Act (SeHA) is a state-level authority to regulate eHealth practices in India.

CLINICAL MODELS FOR TELEPRACTICE
SERVICE DELIVERY IN INDIA

Telepractice can be conducted via three established models:

Synchronous model: This is also known as a direct service model and is used to provide real-time service to patients or clients. Such a service is similar to traditional brick and mortar therapy but conducted in telemode, that is, via videoconferencing software. In this type of service delivery, an SLP can communicate with the client by using target materials and activities.

Asynchronous model: This is also known as the store and forward model where data is stored/captured and sent across to the professional. Using video clippings, voice clips, assessment results, ideas and tips around the intervention plan, are all a part of this model.

Hybrid model: This is a combination of both the synchronous and asynchronous models and the traditional in-person services.

WEB-CONFERENCING

Online teletherapy programme can be provided using three types of web-conferencing options: business class, software-based and public domain.

- *Business class:* Includes purchasing hardware and is typically used at large facilities such as universities or medical centres (e.g., Cisco and Polycom).
- *Software-based:* Includes an encrypted software and an agreement with the practitioner on how the client's privacy is protected (e.g., WebEx, TheraKonnect and VSee).
- *Public domain:* Not always encrypted and private (e.g., FaceTime, Skype and Google Hangouts).

Few of the modes of real-time interaction through applications are:

- Video and text chatting
- Recording (with and without editing capability)
- Screen sharing

- White boards
- Annotation
- Online presentations
- Touch screen
- Interactivity features (e.g., animations, widgets, games, stamps and paintbrush)

THERAKONNECT—INDIA'S FIRST TELEPRACTICE SOFTWARE

TheraKonnect (www.therakonnect.com.)[1] is the first videoconferencing software that was launched in 2018 with an objective to provide a trusted, secure and affordable platform for professionals in India to be able to conduct telepractice using the latest technology (TheraKonnect). The software has enabled many users to start their online work in no time. It is a secure platform to conduct therapies through video mode to the clients worldwide. It is a paid software; they have different plans ranging from single video session to monthly or yearly sessions and the details are available on the website.

Benefits of TheraKonnect

Despite numerous advances in technology, conducting online therapy can be quite a hustle. This is due to lack of availability of an integrated software that can smoothly handle all aspects of communication between clients and therapists. This communication is of three types:

1. *Pre-session communication.* It consists of collecting payments, booking appointments, sending booking confirmations, reminders and giving easy options to reschedule or cancel. Pre-Session communication is essential to maintain healthy relationship with clients by avoiding any confusions and also to ensure revenue coming in smoothly for the practice.
2. *Ongoing-session communication.* This primarily consists of videoconferencing and other associated features such as screen sharing

---

[1] TheraKonnect—Connect better with your clients and start your journey in online therapy. Available at: https://therakonnect.com/ (accessed on 18 December 2019).

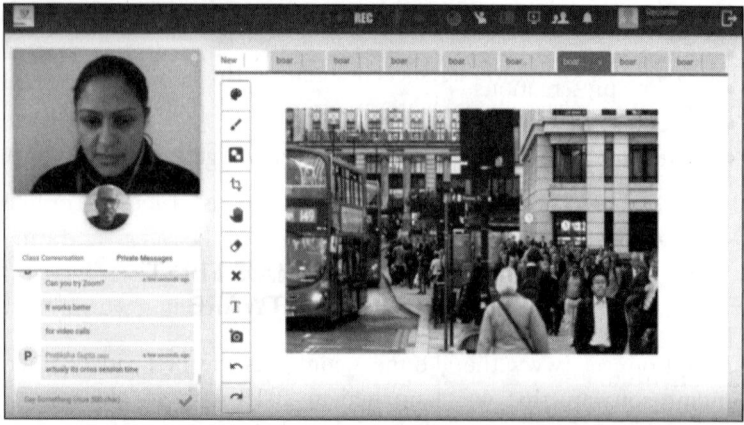

Figure 2.3 *The Screen of TheraKonnect Software is Shared to the Client in a Telepractice Session*

as shown in Figure 2.3 to assist therapists in a therapy session. In traditional videoconferencing solutions like Skype, the interactive features needed for speech therapists are not present. This makes it super difficult for clients to join sessions. Hence, it is important to choose the correct videoconferencing platform.

3. *Post-session communication.* After a session has been successfully completed, it is important to communicate what happened during the session, if any follow ups are needed, session recordings or materials used during the session. This is essential to improve client retention by keeping them apprised and up to date about their therapy progress. Recording of a session is a key differentiator which gives an edge to online therapy over offline therapy. Hence, it is essential to ensure that your therapy platform supports session recordings and provides easy access to them.

TheraKonnect seamlessly handles all three types of communications between a therapist and a client, as far as online therapy is concerned. The platform offers integrated interactive features in the video sessions which enhance therapy outcomes. As a professional one can use TheraKonnect and avoid any technical hustles coming in the way of starting online practice. It is a comprehensive and affordable solution for online speech-language services.

MODIFICATIONS IN ONLINE THERAPY

Telepractice and traditional speech-language therapy are similar in nature but to engage clients better in online sessions, a few modifications are needed.

1. **Facilitator**: A facilitator or e-helper's role is crucial in online speech therapy sessions. The involvement of the caregiver during the session not only helps in conducting the sessions but also directly supplements the parent training/counselling which has a positive effect on the child's development.

2. **Environment**: The environment both at the client's and the therapist's ends should be suitable for therapy. Noise and visual distractions should be kept minimum. Clothes worn by the therapists should be simple and not very distracting.

3. **Seating and posture**: For children with cerebral palsy and other motor deficits, sitting on a high feeding chair with the table/tray in front is most ideal. For children with hyperactivity, seating them in tall chairs with tables in front (so that they are confined to the table/chair) is suitable. The computer should be kept at an optimum distance so that it is neither too far nor too near to the client.

4. **Digital activities**: Using digital resources during therapy has been a breakthrough. Therapists can create customized resources and material depending on the targeted goal and interest of the child. There are various new generation websites which offer engaging games that can be wonderful during the sessions. HearBuilder, Starfall, ABCmouse, PBSkids, Twinkl are great for children.

5. **Apps**: Many apps can be used during the sessions. Google Play Store offers various apps that can be chosen depending on the target activity.

6. **Hands-on activities in online sessions**: Various hands-on activities can be carried out during online therapy sessions. The parents must be instructed about the material requirement in advance. Different crafts, sensory activities, art and colouring, building legos, water play, eating and kitchen-based activities, all can be implemented with careful planning and counselling.

7. **Recording of the sessions**: After taking the consent of the client, online sessions can be recorded to document pre and post-treatment progress.

ADVANTAGES OF TELEPRACTICE OVER CONVENTIONAL SPEECH-LANGUAGE THERAPY

Flexible and Cost-effective

Through telepractice the client can save a lot of time and money spent on travels by the practitioners and clients which reduces the overall cost of the therapy. The clients can also attend therapy sessions even if they are travelling to another city instead of cancelling the sessions. Thus it aids in attending the continued therapy sessions by overcoming many situational barriers like traffic jams, parents being ill or bad weather etc. The adult clients prefer flexibility for the time to manage with their regular jobs, college or any other daily schedules. In addition to these, individuals with physical disabilities or any other health issues can access therapy sessions either from home or office (Crutchley, Alvares and Campbell 2014).

Learning in Natural Environment

The learning behaviour of children is more functional and socially adaptive if it emerges during the natural activities of the day-to-day life (Dunst et al. 2006, 3–10). The child is in his/her natural environment, that is, home, which is the best place for a child to learn language concepts and experiment in his/her functional environment. The learning effectively gets carried over to the day-to-day communication. Whereas in the conventional speech therapy model, the child has to be in the speech-language pathoglogist's geographical area, which is new for the child and causes discomfort and alters his/her natural responses to the stimuli, at least during the initial sessions of the therapy. If the therapy sessions are done at home, parents can be with the child and can monitor his/her activities as well as the progress through the sessions. In some of the conventional speech therapy centres, parents were not allowed inside the room as the child may not follow the instructions of the clinician or may not cooperate for the structured activities planned. However, at the end parents are given an overview of the therapy session and the activities to be performed at home.

Parental Training

In telepractice, especially while dealing with a young child, the SLP will play the role of a coach to the parents. In the family-centred intervention, the parents are educated about the goals and the intervention strategies considered for promoting the skills of the child. The research also shows that the parents learn to get control over the interactions with the child and become the primary facilitator of the child's attempts to communicate (Houston and Behl 2012). Through the coaching process, the parents learn an effective way to facilitate the child's development and growth during everyday learning opportunities (Campbell and Sawyer 2007, 287–305; McWilliam 2010; Rush and Shelden 2011). The parents following the children's lead can have a positive impact on the child's development and learning abilities (Dunst et al. 2006, 3–10).

Joint Monitoring

In telepractice, the therapist and the parents can jointly examine the development of the new skills and competencies and can plan problem-solving strategies. The online sessions can be recorded and viewed later for the parents' reference. The satisfaction of using telepractice service delivery model by SLPs is reported by the clinicians and the parents in western studies (Rose et al. 2000, 101–104; Crutchley, Dudley and Campbell 2010; McCullough 2001, 321–326).

Significant Increase in the Number of Beneficiaries

Telepractice need not be limited to the home-based service, even children in schools/clinics/nursing homes can be screened and treatment services can be provided accordingly. The Indian government encourages for the inclusive education of special children into regular schools, but there are no stringent policies enforced by the government to have an SLP in every school with special kids. Hence, most of the schools do not have an SLP on a regular basis. In India, only 2,500 qualified SLPs are registered with ISHA (Indian Speech and

Hearing Association 2015). In these circumstances, telepractice by SLPs for providing assessment and intervention services can be of great convenience to outreach SLPs' services to a larger portion of population.

CHALLENGES AND ISSUES

There are many challenges involved in telepractice in the field of speech-language pathology such as lack of awareness about the services by SLPs', infrastructure, technology, cultural and language barriers, etc.

Awareness and Acceptance

In India, awareness about the role of an SLP is very less and only a handful of medical and paramedical professionals are aware of the scope of an SLP. Hence, receiving the referrals from other allied professionals is also limited and the clients who directly approach an SLP are scarce. Most of the speech and language disorders need therapy sessions with a frequency of twice or thrice a week over a period of minimum three months to a year or a couple of years. In this scenario, the relocation of the families from remote areas to nearby cities to avail regular therapeutic services from an SLP is difficult. It will be very beneficial if SLPs' services can be available online to reach every person with a disability. However, the major issue is spreading the awareness about the services delivered by the SLPs and accepting the SLP services through telepractice modality.

Infrastructure and Technological Requirements

Connectivity

The Internet connection speed has a significant impact on the quality of video and audio clarity. Expert users opined that the speed of no less than 3 Mbps is needed for optimal connection and screen sharing. Multiple users reduce the speed of the Internet. In case of using high-definition (HD) screen with a dual streaming video presentation or to host multipoint call, higher connection speed no less than 5 Mbps may be required. Lower bandwidth may result in loss of data, jitter and reduced quality of signals for clinical decision making or normal turn-taking in conversational discourse. A minimum bandwidth of 384 Kbps is required to have adequate audio and visual clarity (Jarvis-Selinger et al. 2008, 720–725).

The remote and rural areas do have limited access to Internet facilities. Even though the usage of smartphones and Internet is widespread to remote areas, most of the population residing in remote villages of India still don't have access to high-speed Internet with good connectivity. If the Internet is used by multiple users then onsite technical support may be required.

Videoconferencing Tools

The limited screen size of the mobile phones can restrict the visibility for both the provider and the clients. So it's essential to have a laptop/desktop or a tablet with a good display monitor size, resolution and dual display with built-in/detachable cameras (pan-tilt-zoom and resolution) (Houston 2013). In a school setting, it's preferable to have a camera with wide-angle capabilities with an ability to zoom in and zoom out allowing the SLP to view specific students. These cameras can also be connected to the smartboard to display the SLP image. Peripheral devices, such as recording devices, auxiliary video input equipment for computer interfacing, document cameras (Houston 2013). The software installed on the laptop should support videoconferencing system, whiteboard, document camera, screen sharing and application sharing etc. To work on this software, both the hub and the remote site need to have the software. Initially, this software needs to be purchased and later renewed as required annually. However, there are many free types of software available too for videoconferencing with limited facilities such as Skype, Google Hangouts, Zoom and IMO. Figure 2.4 depicts a speech therapy session using Skype software.

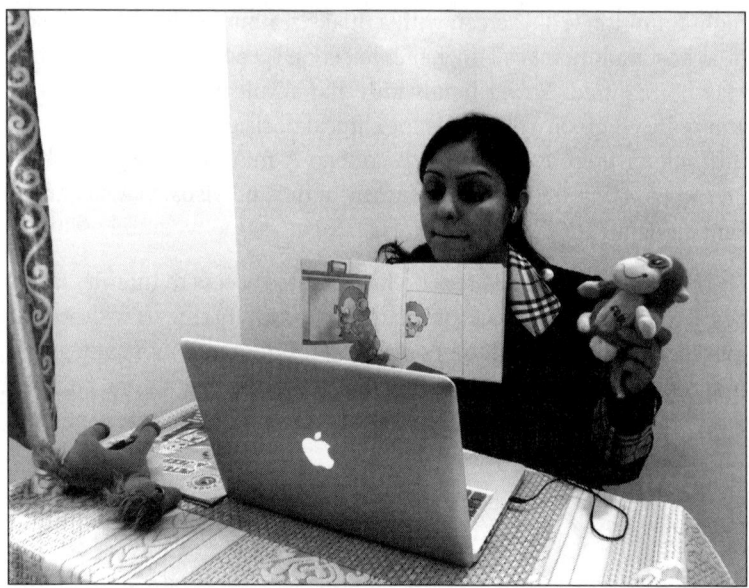

Figure 2.4 *Speech Therapy through Telepractice Model Using TheraKonnect Software*

Privacy and Confidentiality Protocols

Securing the privacy of the client identity and information related to them is utmost important as per the Right to Privacy under Article 21 of the Indian Constitution, there is no federal mandate that manages the rights of protection of data security. Many of the applications used for telepractice services are being conducted through Voice over the Internet Protocol (VoIP) systems such as LINC, iChat, Microsoft Live Meeting and Adobe Connect Now (Watzlaf et al. 2010, 3).

Digital Resources

The digital resources for telepractice are very limited especially in India with multilingual population, it's required to adapt and develop the need-based resources such as flashcards as PowerPoint slides, interactive software consisting of activities like scoring, mobiles and tablets with customized home training applications etc. There are many apps which can be used in general for lexical development. However, disordered specific digital resources need to be developed.

Solutions and Recommendations

There can be a host of recommendations to improve the currently existing model of telepractice in India. Here are some recommendations.

Needs Assessment

To offer a successful telepractice intervention plan to an individual with a speech-language disorder, it is crucial to lay down and develop a plan that addresses objectives such as:

1. The need of the individual or the organization (school or hospital)
2. Awareness-building about the telepractice service model
3. Available infrastructure and technology for telepractice of SLP model programme
4. Plan the approach for documentation
5. Implementation both at home and at school
6. Professional's and caregiver's training agenda
7. Evaluation of the model implementation
8. Adjust the programme as per the requirements (Crutchley, Alvares and Campbell 2014).

Cost-Benefit Analysis

Performing a cost-benefit analysis is an essential component for quality assurance and quality improvement in telepractice. It is better to discuss the client's expenses in detail to attend the conventional model of therapy which includes travel costs, loss of time at work, accommodation costs, if required. Practitioners can ask for if the clients are interested in piloting the videoconferencing session for better understanding of the client. If the client gets motivated to attend the SLP's services through telepractice modality, the SLP evaluates whether the client is familiar with the equipment and the software he/she is planning or has been recommended to use for the telepractice. If a client is technofobic then providing a face to face orientation and demonstration session about the usage of the equipment and the software can put the client at ease.

Information Technology (IT) Support

A telepractising SLP needs constant IT support and collaboration. Such help can be useful in troubleshooting any breakdowns which may occur during online consultation. The collaboration between an off-site SLP and an on-site IT personnel eases the process of technology selection and helps with troubleshooting when issues arise. The practising teleclinician should be aware of the work schedule of the IT personnel. Duties of the IT personnel include ongoing quality assessments, managing firewalls and to ensure enough Internet bandwidth is available during the sessions.

Documentation and Monitoring the Progress and Quality

Monitoring progress and quality of a telepractice programme is imperative. All services should be evaluated for clinical effectiveness and must include client's and telepractitioner's feedback surveys. Professionals should document and record outcomes of the intervention programmes and should make appropriate timely recommendations and referrals. Internet-based frameworks are perfect for telepractice as they allow universal access and association of all the team members.

Documentation of telepractice should include:

1. Date and time of the session
2. Duration of the session
3. Report on any technical issues
4. Goals taken up during the session
5. Activities and responses obtained during the session

Monitoring the progress of the client is an ongoing process. Both the professional and the client should communicate frequently to enhance the overall quality of the telepractice programme. There should be a free flow of information, concerns and questions between them.

Clinical Training

Periodic training of the professional team is crucial for greater results of the therapy programme. The Rehabilitation Council of India (RCI) (2015) approved syllabus for Bachelors in Audiology and Speech-Language Pathology (BASLP) includes a topic on telepractice in audiology and speech-language pathology. Even in post-graduation level, a topic on telepractice is included. In 2015, the RCI approved telepractice model of therapy and documented the scope of an SLP in evaluation and therapy. Besides, the private firm 1SpecialPlace conducts short term and advanced online training courses for beginners on telepractice. 1SpecialPlace has also set up a networking and collaboration group for telepractioners on Facebook[2] called The Telerehab Club (The Telerehab Club). By expanding the knowledge about the telepractice among students pursuing degree courses, can ease and encourage telepractice among upcoming professionals. Following aspects must be included in the training:

1. Advantages and drawbacks of telepractice
2. Documenting data in standardized method
3. Importance of professional certification
4. Networking with other tele professionals
5. Planning for teletherapy sessions
6. Techniques and behavioural management approaches
7. Communication with team members and caregivers
8. Resources and materials used in the intervention
9. Collaboration with IT professionals

Providing Security Connections

Computers used for telepractice should have a secure firewall and an updated antivirus software package installed. These security methods help in reducing the chances of a virus attack and maintain the privacy of the client's information (Boisvert et al. 2012, 11–24). Most of the

---

[2] The Telerehab Club—Network for Teletherapists from across the World. Available at: https://www.facebook.com/groups/636251976562701/(accessed on 18 December 2019).

videoconferencing applications are based on a server and the conversations are routed through a central server. The signals passed through some of these systems are automatically encrypted to avoid hacking and ensure confidentiality. Few VoIP services request for an additional fee for encryption of the signals. It is better to have a knowledge of how the service provider is handling the data. Do they store the data or just pass through it (Crutchley, Alvares and Campbell 2014)?

Obtaining Consent

Providing telepractice model of therapy by following ethical guidelines safeguards the clinician and facilitates quality services to the client. Gathering informed consent of the client, to initiate the tele-intervention plan, is very important. This should include the following:

1. Providing a description of the technology to be used
2. Discussing the nature of service delivery
3. Counselling about the differences between telepractice and traditional therapy

CASE VIGNETTES

Client with Dysarthria

Background Information

A male client, aged 36 years, reported having difficulty in communicating with his limited abilities to speak followed by a stroke. In addition to the loss of speech, he also had feeding and swallowing difficulties. This had a significant impact on his profession as he was a senior consultant dealing with many clients on a daily basis. He could not continue regular speech therapy session due to practical issues related to the job, travelling and his health conditions. The client started searching for speech therapy services online. He found 1SpecialPlace through Google search engine and enquired for the services. He was offered to attend a free trial session prior to enrolling for speech therapy to understand the possibilities of telespeech therapy services followed by an assessment. The client was convinced and enrolled for therapy with a frequency of two sessions per week and each session lasting for an hour.

Tele-assessment

Prior to starting the session, the client was instructed to have a high speed Internet connection with good quality microphones and headphones. The speech therapist also emailed the materials that were required for the speech and language assessment and the client was also requested to email the medical reports to the speech therapist prior to assessment. The client was assessed using TheraKonnect software.

The detailed case history was collected by the therapist followed by informal observations and clinical correlation with a formal test battery. During the interaction, the therapist noticed that the client was able to deliver the content effectively however speech intelligibility was poor. The client was able to follow the therapist's instructions and respond accordingly. As the client comprehended well, he did not require any assistance from the caretaker to attend online speech therapy sessions.

Oro peripheral examination. The appearance of oral structures was normal. Functions of structures were assessed by systematic instructions to the client. Lip puckering, holding the button with the lips tied to a thread, alternate retraction and protrusion of lips were performed. Movements of the tongue, velum, jaw and vegetative skills were also evaluated.

Formal Tests

Western Aphasia Battery (Kertesz 1982). The results indicated aphasia quotient (AQ) 97.4 suggesting the absence of aphasia.

Frenchay Dysarthria Assessment (Enderby 1980, 165–173). Based on the findings, client was diagnosed with dysarthria secondary to stroke.

Intervention

The client started up with online speech therapy sessions for a duration of 45 minutes conducted thrice a week and the targeted goals were briefly explained. Material required for online sessions were mailed by the clinician prior to the session.

Long term goal. To improve his overall speech intelligibility for effective communication.

Short term goal. To improve articulatory movements and precision in the production, coordination with the respiration during the conversation.

Activities of Online Speech Therapy Sessions

Respiratory and phonatory coordination. Thoracoabdominal breathing is demonstrated and encouraged to do while phonation. Feedback is provided to improve his maximum phonation duration and mean length of utterance were monitored.

Articulatory movements and precision in production. Tongue exercises and lip strengthening exercises were also demonstrated and articulatory drilling was performed for the distorted consonants. Various words were also dictated and used in sentence forms and access was given to the client to use the whiteboard as shown in Figure 2.5.

Monitoring progress and providing feedback. Recordings of sessions were done and mailed to the client which served as the feedback.

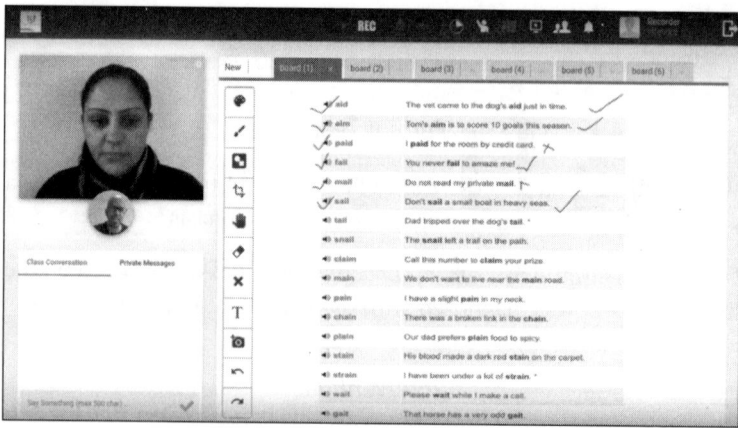

Figure 2.5 *The Client Using a Whiteboard in the TheraKonnect Software*

Videos on performing the exercises and words for articulatory drilling were also displayed on the screen, shared through TheraKonnect.

Connectivity issues during online sessions. Occasionally network connectivity was poor at both client's and provider's hub. During those times the clinician would have a telephonic conversation with the client and provided guidance for troubleshooting. If a network issue existed longer, then recorded materials with detailed instructions were sent to the client via email and the session was rescheduled.

Progress of the Online Therapy

The progress was observed after 12 sessions and client was also able to generalize the improvement to the outside environment. Overall, the client was satisfied by the online speech therapy services of 1SpecialPlace and he was able to start up with his work after 3 months of intensive speech therapy services and was able to generalize the tips and ideas provided by the speech therapist in his day-to-day practice. The progress in a few components of Frenchay Dysarthria Assessment (FDA) analysis is depicted in Figure 2.6.

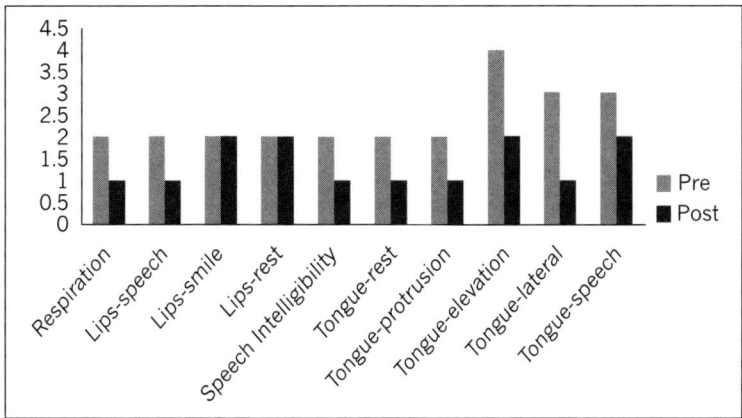

Figure 2.6 *Frenchay Dysarthria Assessment (FDA) Scores of Pre- and Post-therapy Evaluation*

Score 1 depicts no abnormalities in articulatory functions and as the score increases the severity of abnormality increases and most severe is related to score 5.

Recommendations. Client XYZ was recommended to continue the sessions once a week for a period of 6 months and he was explained about the need for reassessment that was carried out after 6 months and the findings revealed improved intelligibility during conversation as he was able to maintain a good respiratory control along with the adequate lip and tongue movements necessary for good speech. Thus, online therapy had a great impact on the client and helped him to continue his professional career in a smooth manner and he was recommended for follow-ups for every 6 months along with the continuation of the home-based activities suggested by the clinician.

2.2 Client with Cerebral Palsy

Background Information

A child, aged four years and six months reported having a history of preterm cesarean section delivery and delayed birth cry. Her birth weight was below average. Parents also reported seizures soon after birth until 3 years of age. The developmental history reveals that her motor milestones and speech milestones were significantly delayed. She was diagnosed with delayed speech and language development with cerebral palsy (dystonia) by a multidisciplinary team consisting of an SLP, a physiotherapist and a psychologist.

The child is under physical therapy care since she was born. She started traditional speech therapy but couldn't continue as both the parents were working and they found managing school and physical therapy very difficult. The child started online speech therapy twice a week at 1SpecialPlace. The parents were accessing intervention from their home.

Tele-assessment

The child was assessed using TheraKonnect software. Prior to detailed assessment the parents were instructed to have the materials such as pictures of fruits, animals and a few more toys ready for the tele-diagnostic therapy session. The assessment involved a detailed case history, parents' interview, informal observation of the child carrying out various activities such as (a) conversation (b) interaction of the child and parent (c) reaction to questions, rhymes, simple instructions and (d) play. Vegetative skills of blowing, sucking, biting and chewing were observed using appropriate test material. The formal test used was Receptive & Expressive Emergent Language Scale (REELS) to evaluate the child's language abilities and test administration was done almost an hour.

Examples of activities during the assessment: Through TheraKonnect software, various pictures were screen shared with the parents and the mother was instructed to make the child match the desired object with a picture. Various social reinforcements (e.g., clap) that included both the visual and the auditory messages were delivered by the clinician after each correct response. The clinician also provided access to the parents on a whiteboard and encouraged the child to draw pictures on it along with the mother. Rhymes were also presented to the child and the mother was encouraged to perform the actions along with the clinician. The entire session was video recorded by the clinician and watched later to evaluate in detail. Prelinguistic skills like eye contact, attention, concentration, sitting tolerance and compliance were good as observed.

Speech assessment was done by instructing the child to phonate the vowels a/e/i/o/u as long as she can and the mother was asked to draw the line on the whiteboard provided by the software to encourage the child phonation. The child was able to phonate for 3–4 seconds. The child was also evaluated for the phonetic and phonological abilities.

Oro peripheral examination (OPE): OPE revealed the normal appearance and restricted movements of the articulators affecting the vegetative skills along with the speech skills. There was also incoordination between the respiratory, phonatory and articulatory systems resulting in the inadequate intra oral breath pressure during speech production.

Language abilities: Receptive language skills were below average as she exhibited difficulty in understanding complex inclusion/exclusion concepts, multi-level sequencing, conditionals and temporal concepts. Expressive language skills were poor as she struggled to produce word combinations to form phrases. Communication had been mainly via simple and two-word approximations and gestures. Overall her language abilities were just below 2 years of age. Gard Gilman Gorman Speech and Language Development chart was also used to evaluate the child in detail for phonology, semantics, play, syntax-morphology and pragmatics. This test also indicated a significant overall delay in language abilities. The child also had a very low volume while speaking and her communication was mostly non-verbal with strangers.

Multidisciplinary team evaluation and provisional diagnosis. The child was also evaluated by the physiotherapist and the psychologist along with the SLP. The child was diagnosed as having delayed speech and language development with cerebral palsy.

Teletherapy

Long-term goal: To improve the child's speech and language skills for effective communication.

Short-term goals: Receptive language skills, expressive language skills and speech skills are part of the short-term goals.

Receptive language skills: To improve the understanding of 1 step unrelated commands, lexical categories, and simple stories without prompts.

Expressive language skills: To improve the usage of functional words, answer simple questions using mono or disyllabic words and start using an AAC app (augmentive and alternative communication app) more consistently while expressing different needs. To improve social skills such as turn-taking, greeting, topic initiation, etc.

Speech skills: To improve the coordination between respiratory, phonatory, resonatory and articulatory systems. Work on the production of b/p/m sounds in various positions.

List of Few Activities Carried Out during Telepractice

Learning lexical categories. To improve the understanding of lexical categories www.starfall.com was screen shared and the child was encouraged to match the projected items with the objects along with the mother.

Comprehending simple commands. To improve the understanding of simple one-step unrelated commands, initial demonstration of the commands was carried out by the clinician followed by the mother and PowerPoint pictures were presented and screen shared in the session.

Mean length utterance. To improve the MLU finger thumb analogy strategy was demonstrated to the parent and she was modelled to train the child followed by the clinician (one finger-one word).

Pragmatic skills and effective communication. The mother was encouraged to make a scrapbook that includes various events in the child's life and conversation building was done by reinforcing child to initiate about each picture. Parents were explained about the effective usage of *Jellow app* for effective communication beyond the therapy settings and generalize in day-to-day activities.

Oromotor and vegetative skills. These skills were targeted by coaching the parent and demonstration of the task. The mother was explained the use of homemade manometer for promoting blowing skills. Pictures were also shared to prompt for oromotor exercises, as shown in Figure 2.7.

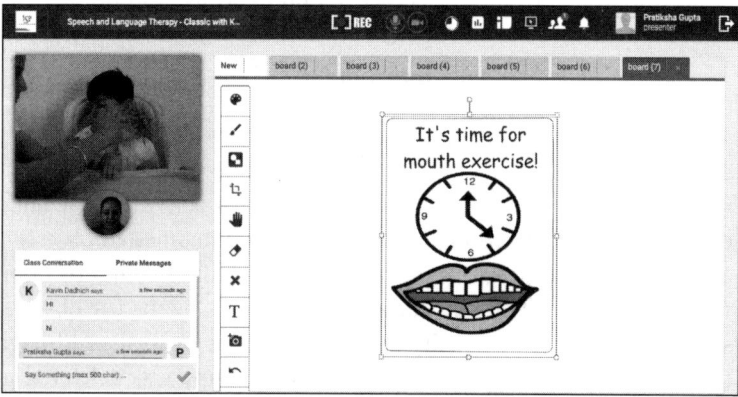

Figure 2.7 *Prompting in Telepractice Model of Speech Therapy for Oromotor Exercises*

Documentation and Quality Maintenance

After every three months, the video recordings were presented to the parents and were discussed about the generalization of new skills and competencies achieved by the child. The therapist was also in regular contact with the child and monitored the child's progress by identifying the adjustments required for the plan. Thus, online therapy services promoted enhanced family and parent-therapist relationships and parental competency of the child. The mother worked as a partner with the clinician and was involved in each step of the child's progress.

2.3 Client with Autism Spectrum Disorder

Background Information

A child aged 11 years, male, had a history of delayed speech and language. He was diagnosed to be on the Autism Spectrum Disorder at the age of four. He has been receiving regular intervention including applied behaviour analysis, remedial academic help, occupational therapy and language intervention ever since. He had age-inappropriate social language and pragmatic skills.

Baseline evaluation revealed below-average pragmatic language skills, poor decision making and inappropriate social skills. Receptive and expressive language skills were found to be age-appropriate.

Intervention

The intervention included three sessions every week. The duration of each session was halved as compared to traditional therapy sessions as the child lost focus and attention with longer activities. The child exhibited poor motivation and compliance and manifested obsessive and narrowed interests for activities and stimuli. The intervention was aimed at improving his social language skills by the use of social stories which were personalized according to his interests. Although the child's native language was Hindi, the therapy was delivered in English. Target goals also included phonics and improving reading fluency in English language as shown in Figure 2.8. Improving language

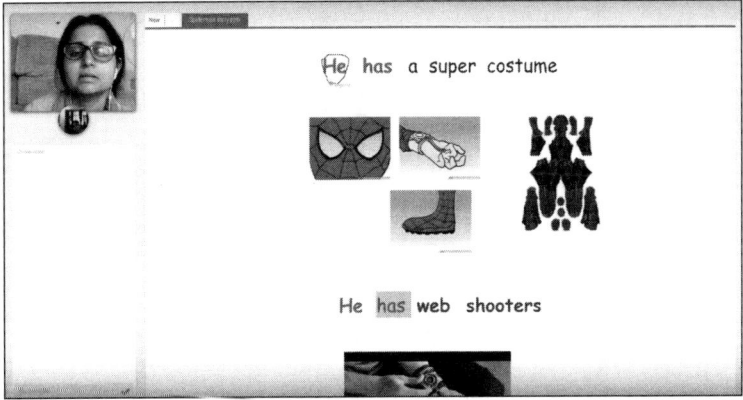

Figure 2.8 *Telepractice to Improve English Fluency*

expression in English was also a target. Each session was followed by consistent functional practice guidelines to the mother who was sent an email with the session summary and simple carryover activities to be carried out at home as shown in Figure 2.9.

Speech and Language Outcomes

Results of qualitative analysis between baseline and post-intervention show a significant improvement in reading high-frequency words and also a few sight words. He can now read level 1 book related to his interests. He shows better motivation to read and have conversations in English. Pragmatic skills, social appropriateness, reading fluency, and compliance. The progress is ongoing with using socially appropriate language and showing better compliance with persons in his family. The mother reported satisfactory results from the qualitative survey which was carried out.

DISCUSSION

Telepractice in the field of speech-language pathology is still in the budding stage in India. Limited numbers of SLPs working in India are indulged in telepractice for providing assessment and treatment

Dear Parents,

Thank You for being there and sharing details and ideas during the session.

Please find attached material for reference. If you have any concerns or if some activity is not working out for Tanish, please let me know. Please share the videos as discussed. Also, I would encourage you to take photographs of Tanish :

- Doing daily routines
- Involved in the activities we discussed
- Outside places

HomeWork:

1. Pretend Play with Balloons - Draw a picture of an animal and use it for pretend play. For example, make the dog walk, run, jump, give it a bath, feed it etc.

2. Hitting the balloon with a bat

3. Cognitive Play: Stick pictures of pairs of things that go together, for example, socks and shoes, plate and food, shirt and pant, bed and pillow. Stick these pictures on different corners or walls of the room. Lead your child to associate them together by sticking it next to each other.
Another variation of this activity is to get 4-5 household items, sit in front of him, label them all and then lead him to put it away in their respective places. For example, put the toothbrush away in the bathroom etc.

4. Teach theme-based vocabulary to Tanish. Examples:
Food Items
Art and craft vocabulary
Outside places
Inside home

We will review 15 days later.

Best Wishes,

Figure 2.9 *Screenshot of the Email Written to the Parents with the Goals and Activities*

services. A colossal country like India, with 1.34 billion population and limited SLPs, is in deadly need of speech therapy services through telepractice model of service delivery. Currently, this is one of the best ways to extend speech therapy services to the populations in remote areas as technology has reached the corners of India. The Indian government, in fact, started e-Hospital services and DISHA (Ingle, 2017) to enable digital sharing of health records across hospitals and clinics. To promote and regulate the standards of 'e-health services', the Indian government developed NeHA. Specific to online speech therapy services, the AIISH is the government organization providing speech therapy services through telepractice mode. Apart from this, there are very few private firms such as 1SpecialPlace, SRMC, Bhartiya Vidyapeeth etc., delivering speech therapy services through telepractice model. In 2017, AIISH published policies for telepractice mode of speech therapy services focusing on various administrative, clinical, technical and ethical issues.

In spite of having the digitally literate population in India still speech therapy services through telepractice mode are limited. Yashaswini and Rao (2018) conducted a survey and based on the reports from the service providers and receivers; the authors summarized the potential barriers to telepractice. The service providers report that there are many technical barriers such as technophobia to use videoconferencing software, other related technology to interact during the sessions as screen sharing, whiteboard, etc. Even constant access to high-speed Internet (Yashaswini and Rao 2018, 1–8), lack of awareness among the public regarding speech therapy, acceptance of telepractice and inadequate training to SLP's in telepractice are some of the issues contributing to the limited services through telepractice in India. Concerns about client confidentiality are expressed, and lack of direct feedback and environmental distractions at client end are also reported as challenges in telepractice delivery in India (Yashaswini and Rao 2018, 1–8).

To overcome the hurdles in providing speech therapy services through telepractice model, the initial step is to refine the skills of SLPs to work on telepractice model. In 2015, the RCI approved the scope of the SLPs through telepractice modality (S. Rep. No. 2–6/RCI/2015, 2015) and accordingly, the syllabus for professional training also included topics on telepractice. Even a private firm 1SpecialPlace is also conducting a short term online training course on telepractice. By expanding the knowledge of telepractice among students pursuing the degree, can ease and encourage telepractice among upcoming professionals.

In addition to the training to service providers (SLPs) the service receivers (clients) also require support, especially related to the use of technology. Clients can be provided constant guidance and if required, an assistant too with technical knowledge about the equipment and software used for telepractice to facilitate the therapy in the initial sessions. Other practical issues like networking problems can be handled if the videoconferencing system has an option to store and forward function. Most of the Indian families cannot offer to purchase the equipment required for the telepractice from home. In such cases, asynchronous or hybrid clinical model of telepractice can be encouraged. The client can send video and audio clips of communication act to the therapist for analysis through public Internet facilities or mobiles. Based on the requirements with respect to the disorders, occasional face-to-face interaction sessions can be planned while taking regular therapy through telepractice modality. The training materials can be provided to the client for the related activities to achieve the goals prior to the telepractice sessions. If there is any technological interruption then recorded audio or video clips of the planned activities can be sent by the caregiver to the SLP for further analysis and guidance. A study by Carey et al. (2012) evaluated the efficacy of three adolescent participants attending therapy over Skype once in a week and sending the audio clips for later review. The results revealed that group mean reduction of 83 per cent of syllables stuttered from pretherapy to entry to maintenance for three clients.

Research on the efficacy of telepractice model to deliver SLP services in India is still evolving. In India, the first case study published on the efficacy of tele-intervention in the field of speech-language pathology is by Goswami, Bhutada and Jayachandran (2012). They have studied the efficacy of speech and language therapy delivered through telemodel through Skype for a client with Broca's Aphasia. They found significant improvement in expression, repetition, naming and memory skills and concluded that telepractice can be an effective mode of therapy. In abroad, the telepractice by SLPs is well-documented efficacy based approach (Carey et al. 2012, 370–380).

The social and cultural differences need to be considered and adapted to provide SLP services through telepractice mode. For instance, providing the digital materials used can be more specific to the clients' needs. There are several general apps HearBuilder, Starfall, ABCmouse, PBSkids, Twinkl which can be used to work on developing lexical categories. However, disorder or skill-specific digital resources developed in other countries such as Constant Therapy (2017), Aphasia Corner (2017) and Boardmaker Online (2017) need to be developed in India (Rao and Yashaswini 2019, 67). AIISH developed digital materials and are available in the telecentre and helpline websites dedicated to the telepractice services. There is a range of short videos on disorders, self-evaluation checklists, home training materials, tele-orientation videos and success stories are available (Rao and Yashaswini 2019, 67).

Yashaswini and Rao (2018) recommended for validation of digital resources in various Indian languages, conducting empirical studies focusing on mode of service delivery in telepractice (virtual or hybrid, face-to-face), protecting the privacy on e-platforms, revising code of ethics for SLPs, cost-benefit and risk analysis can have a significant impact to have surge in telepractice in India. Application of telepractice can range from primary prevention (public education) to tertiary rehabilitation services such as teleguidance to caregivers, tele-assessment, and tele-intervention in India (Rao and Yashaswini 2019, 67).

FUTURE DIRECTIONS

Manpower development. To provide services to 26.8 million of the population with disabilities (India Census Data 2011), there is a severe shortage of SLPs. The application of telepractice using technological advancements offers effective solutions to this challenge in future. Hence, the SLPs need to be trained in telepractice. The policies need to get stringent and every graduate in speech-language pathology should have practical exposure and it should be reflected in the clinical practicum certificate.

Efficacy research studies. The efficacy of telepractice in India needs to be researched. These kinds of studies can enhance the use of telepractice by SLPs and even acceptance for telepractice will improve among the clients too.

Digital resource development. There is a need for the development of client-specific and need-based resources. It is challenging to use digital resources just based on the English language in India as most of the children with speech disorders will be provided speech and language therapy in their native language. Hence, digital resources need to be developed in various Indian languages.

Encouraging teletherapy. The government organizations and private firms can slowly shift from face-to-face therapy sessions to the hybrid model of teletherapy where initial sessions are face-to-face sessions and later are based on telepractice model. This model aids in developing trust on SLPs and continuing therapy in telepractice model. Later, it is possible to shift from a hybrid model to the synchronous model of telepractice. The government has to take initiatives to provide telepractice model of therapy at every government hospital to serve the people residing in remote areas and economically poor. Including SLP services through the current government online health platforms such as e-health and provide information related to the prevention of communication disorders through mHealth services. The government need to fund the infrastructure required to avail the speech therapy services to the clients exhibiting restricted mobility. Even health insurances policies can include the speech-language pathology services for insurance coverage.

Multidisciplinary telepractice services. A common platform needs to be created where the clients are evaluated and the reports are shared. This can be accessible to various health care professionals dealing with the particular client and there should be a provision to interact and plan the intervention programme. The follow-up and post-treatment evaluations also need to be documented on the same platform and should be made available to the health care professionals handling that particular client.

Technological Advancements. There is a need to develop simple software with ease of operation to interact during the videoconferencing and share the documents, screens or videos. The Internet connectivity needs to be improved especially in the remote areas of the city limits.

Privacy and Security Issues. The security of the freely available videoconferencing software packages need to be improved. Through smartphones, video calling and videoconferencing are possible, using software such as Skype, OoVoo, WiCall, fring, MobileVoip and Tango. However the privacy and encryption concerns are limiting their usage in health care.

Virtual self-help groups anchored by professionals. Virtual self-help groups for person-to-person support anchored by a professional through Facebook, Twitter, technical blogs and similar social media sites would also serve as a good prospect to build up a network. This mode of service delivery calls for multilingual resources for Indian population shared across centres and individuals, of course with terms and conditions that help to systematize our services.

CONCLUSION

Technology, healthcare and education have converged to give birth to telepractice which is a revolutionary approach to treat patients with communication disorders. India is gripped with a national shortage of professionals and telepractice offers great benefits by making services accessible and affordable to millions. As opposed to internationally prevalent telepractice methods, which are extravagant and use high-quality videoconferencing dedicated units both at the provider and at the receiver's end, Indian population would rather benefit from exploring Internet-based platforms and resources for telediagnostics and intervention. Although this method of service delivery is picking up momentum, we still have challenges of awareness, acceptance, knowledge, training, research, standardization, licensing, ethical supervision and funds to scale it up at a level where it is a preferred choice for everyone. As tele practitioners, we know how beneficial this is, what has to be done, how it has to be done, why it has to be done and so now, it's just a question of why not.

APPENDIX A

Table 2A.1 *A Sample of the Format Used to Plan the Goals and Activities*

Skills	Baseline	Goals
Reading English— reading fluency, reading comprehension, and answering questions	Reluctant to read English, reads CVC words. Doesn't phonetically sound out words and tries to guess lengthy words.	To motivate and improve reading fluency by: • Introducing high-frequency words • Reading sight words • Teach decoding phonetically tricky words—diagraphs such as 'oo', ea' and split diagraphs such as 'a-e, u-e as in make, blue etc. • Work up to reading sentences and answering related questions.
Social-pragmatic language skills	Has difficulty understanding other person's perspective— finds topic maintenance challenging Has difficulty controlling anger— blaming, does not use appropriate language to express his dislikes Has an obsession for LEGO toys—becomes a compulsive topic to maintain his interest in learning activities	Use social story and conversation strips to remediate these issues

APPENDIX B

Patient Testimonials

1. My son has been receiving online speech therapy from Mrs XYZ from 1SpecialPlace, I am glad to let you know that he is making good progress in his pre-linguistic skills. Mrs XYZ is very expressive while

demonstrating actions and words which keeps the child engaged in the activity and enhances the learning process. She plans the activities of the session in a way that includes a step by step approach towards the development of speech and language. She discusses with the parents and provides study material as per the requirement of the child. I am hopeful that, with continued online speech therapy lessons my son is going to make remarkable progress in areas of speech and language.

— Mother of an 18-year-old with ASD

2. My son has completed 10 sessions. There is a tremendous change in his speech. Earlier, he used to speak very few words. But with the sessions, he is using 3–4 words sentences already. He is four years old. We used to worry a lot. But now knowing there is nothing wrong with him, which every parent could understand, is the biggest relief. He is improving with each session. We thank 1SpecialPlace which made speech therapy possible from our home. We recommend it to every parent who is concerned about their child's speech. Thank you 1SpecialPlace!

—Mother of a 4-year-old child with Expressive Language Delay

REFERENCES

1SpecialPlace for speech and language enrichment 2018. Available at: http://www.1specialplace.com (accessed on 18 December 2019)..

American Speech-Language-Hearing Association. 2004. *Preferred Practice Patterns For The Profession of Speech-Language Pathology* {Preferred Practice Patterns}. Available at: http://www.asha.org/policy (accessed on 18 December 2019).

Boisvert, M., N. Hall, M. Andrianopoulos, and J. Chaclas. 2012. 'The Multi-Faceted Implementation of Telepractice to Service Individuals with Autism.' *International Journal of Telerehabilitation*, 4 (2): 11–24.

Campbell, P. H., and L. B. Sawyer. 2007. 'Supporting Learning Opportunities in Natural Settings Through Participation-Based Services.' *Journal of Early Intervention*, 29 (4): 287–305.

Carey, B., S. O'Brian, M. Onslow, A. Packman, and R. Menzies. 2012. 'Webcam delivery of the Camperdown Program for Adolescents Who Stutter: A Phase I trial.' *Language, Speech, and Hearing Services in Schools*, 43 (3): 370–380.

Crutchley, S., R. L. Alvares, and M. Campbell. 2014. 'Getting Started: Building a Successful Telepractice Program.' In *Telepractice in Speech-Language Pathology*, edited by K. T. Houston, 51–81. San Diego, CA: Plural Publishing.

Crutchley, S., Dudley, and M. Campbell. 2010. 'Assessment of Articulation by Telepractice: A Pilot Study.' *Presented at the ASHA Convention*, Philadelphia, PA, 18 November 2010.

Darkins, A. W., and M. A. Cary. 2000. *Telemedicine and Telehealth: Principles, Policies, Performances and Pitfalls*. New York: Springer.

Dunst, C. J., M. B. Bruder, C. M. Trivette, and D. W. Hamby. 2006. 'Everyday Activity Settings, Natural Learning Environments, and Early Intervention Practices.' *Journal of Policy and Practice in Intellectual Disabilities*, 3 (1): 3–10.

Enderby, Pamela. 1980. 'Frenchay Dysarthria Assessment.' *British Journal of Disorders of Communication* 15 (3): 165–173.

Goswami, S. P., A. Bhutada, and K. Jayachandran. 2012. 'Telepractice in a Person with Aphasia.' *Journal of the All India Institute of Speech & Hearing*, 31: 159–167.

Houston, K. T. 2013. *Telepractice in Speech-Language Pathology*. San Diego, CA: Plural Publishing.

Houston, K. T. and D. Behl. 2012. *Using Telepractice to Improve Outcomes for Children with Hearing Loss and Their Families*. In *EHDI E-Book*, edited by L. Schmeltz. Available at: http://www.infanthearing.org/ehdi-ebook/index.html (accessed on 18 December 2019).

Indian Speech and Hearing Association (ISHA). 2015. The Professional. Available at: https://www.ishaindia.org.in/professional.html/ (accessed on 15 August 2017).

Ingle, Manas. 2017. India: DISHA—The Future Direction of Digital Health Information in India. 2017. Available at: http://www.mondaq.com/india/x/728652/Healthcare/DISHA+The+Future+Direction+Of+Digital+Health+Information+In+India (accessed on 18 December 2019).

Jarvis-Selinger, S., E. Chan, R. Payne, K. Plohman, and K. Ho. 2008. 'Clinical Telehealth Across the Disciplines: Lessons Learned.' *Telemedicine and e-Health*, 14: 720–725.

Kertesz, A. 1982. *Western Aphasia Battery (WAB)*. San Antonio, TX: The Psychological Corporation.

McCullough, A. 2001. 'Viability and Effectiveness of Teletherapy for Preschool Children with Special Needs.' *International Journal of Language & Communication Disorders*, 36 (S1): 321–326.

McWilliam, R. A. 2010. *Working with Families of Young Children with Special Needs*. New York: Guilford Press.

Mohan, H. S., A. Anjum, and P. K. Rao. 2017. 'A Survey of Telepractice in Speech-Language Pathology And Audiology in India'. *International Journal of Telerehabilitation*, 9 (2): 69.

NSSO GOI. 2002. Ministry of Statistics and Programme Implementation, National Sample Survey Office. Available at: http://www.mospi.gov.in. (accessed on 27 February 2019).

Office of the Registrar General & Census Commissioner, India. 2011. India Census Data. Available at: http://www.censusindia.gov.in/2011-Common/CensusData2011.html (accessed on 03 March 2019).

Rao, P. K. S., and R. Yashaswini. 2019. 'Telepractice in Speech-Language Pathology and Audiology: Prospects and Challenges.' *Journal of Indian Speech Language & Hearing Association*, 32 (2): 67.

Rehabilitation Council of India. 2015. 'Scope of Practice in Audiology and Speech-Language Pathology.' Available at: https://kalpagiri.wordpress. com/2017/01/12/rci-news-scope-of-practice-in-audiology-and-speech-language-pathology/ (accessed on 18 December 2019)

Rose, D. A. D., S. Furner, A. Hall, K. Montgomery, E. Katsavras, and P. Clarke. 2000. 'Videoconferencing for Speech and Language Therapy in Schools.' *BT Technology Journal*, 18 (1): 101–104.

Rush, Dathan D. and M'Lisa L. Shelden. 2011. *The Early Childhood Coaching Handbook*. Baltimore, MD: Paul H. Brookes.

Savithri, S. R. and M. Jayaram. 2003. 'Professional Services of AIISH Graduates: International Scenario.' *Unpublished project report* funded by AIISH Research Fund, Mysore.

Telecom Regulatory Authority of India. 2014. Highlights on Telecom Subscription; 28th February, 2014. Available at: http://www.trai.gov.in/sites.default/files/PR-TSD-Feb-23_04_14.pdf (accessed on 15 June 2016).

TheraKonnect—Connect better with your clients and start your journey in online therapy. Available at: https://therakonnect.com/(accessed on 18 December 2019).

The Telerehab Club—Network for Teletherapists from across the World. Available at: https://www.facebook.com/groups/636251976562701/(accessed on 18 December 2019).

Watzlaf, V. J. M., S. Moeini, L. Matusow, and P. Firouzan. 2010. 'VoIP for Telerehabilitation: A Risk Analysis for Privacy, Security and HIPAA Compliance: Part I.' *International Journal of Telerehabilitation*, 3 (1): 3.

Yashaswini, R. and P. K. Rao. 2018. 'Tele Speech-Language Pathology and Audiology in India-A Short Report.' *Journal of the International Society for Telemedicine and eHealth*, 6 (1): e19 (1–8).

Utility of Apps in Speech and Language Therapy

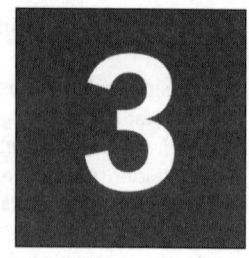

Abhishek B. P. and
Abdulaziz Saleh Almudhi

INTRODUCTION

Communication is the behaviour that makes human social being, thus, demarcating human communication from the form of communication adapted by other species in general. However, this behaviour seems to be meaningful when the sender transmits a message through icons, non-verbal gestures or verbal mode and those messages conveyed should be understood with ease by the receiver. Owens (2006) defined communication as 'exchange of ideas between a sender and a receiver'. Communication has the virtue of using multimodal cues. In spite of that, majority of communication is attained through speech. Consequently, the process enhanced by the use of facial expressions, gestures, eye gaze and so on.

Albeit, there are various modes through which communication can occur. However, a larger part of communication is directly dependent on speech and language process. Whereas, speech sounds are combined in various ways to form language that was used for verbal communication. In general, the aforementioned process becomes critical in all human species. Consequently, these processes are affected in various individuals due to a wide variety of factors. Thus, addressing these individual's communication skills becomes imperative and illuminating the knowledge about thus becomes the pivotal role of a speech-language pathologist (SLP).

An individual's deficits pertaining to communication are termed to have communication disorder in general. A communication disorder is a broad and generic term; it can refer to speech and language disorders. Speech disorders can be referred to disorders concerning voice, fluency and articulation while the language disorders can be classified into child language and adult language disorders. However, these have widespread effects in various domains such as social, emotional well-being and cognition (McKinnon, Sharynne and Sheena 2007, 05–15).

The profiles exhibited by clients with a communication disorder may seem heterogeneous. For instance, children exhibiting disorders such as hearing impairment, intellectual disability, cerebral palsy, can exhibit differences in the profile as the underlying causative itself is different. In the same line, even while rehabilitating aphasia, the causative conditions should be taken into account as the manifestation of language deficits is directly dependent on it. In certain conditions, the causative factor itself may be idiopathic or these factors may combine to complicate the issue further. Thus, rehabilitating these individuals through effective protocol becomes imperative. At this juncture, it is vital to explore various paradigms that can be used to treat individuals with communication disorders. In general, they are paradigms which are designed to proliferate communication skills, through traditional low-tech technique which primarily uses pen and paper. In contrast, delivering therapies using technologies (apps) has received a greater interest in professionals treating individuals with a communication disorder.

UTILITY OF APPS IN COMMUNICATION DISORDER

Apps have revolutionized health care professionals, due to their widespread effects in the field of communication disorders. Along with, other allied medical conditions too. Apps can be used for all communication disorders. The apps can be used for stimulus presentation, employing materials required for therapy like flashcards, pictures, and teaching the concepts. These apps are very user-friendly; thus, in turn, can be used during in-home training and enable easy access to therapy materials. It is feasible to the clinician or the parents to rely on these apps as all the information is available on a single platform and is available at the fingertips. The basic understanding of apps would be a pre-requisite in understanding the utility of apps in communication disorders.

'App' is an acronym for the word *application*. It refers to a software program configured for performing a specific action. The term app can refer to a mobile or a computer application. Apps can be installed or downloaded from platforms or app stores. Some of the apps can be retrieved free while some have to be purchased. While the traditional apps designed for desktop or laptop is to be installed, the apps designed for mobile phones can be downloaded directly. The apps are assumed to be much cheaper compared to software's installed on desktop and laptop primarily because they are less advanced and require relatively limited resources for the development.

Apps can be classified as native apps, the utility apps and hybrid apps, based on the development. Native apps are developed exclusively for a specific platform. Example for native apps is an app which is developed for the iOS platform and cannot be retrieved on an Android or a Symbian platform. Web apps are stored on a remote server. A browser is required for the web-based app to run. The hybrid app combines elements of both web app and native app. The cost of development is assumed too high for native app followed by hybrid and a web-based app.

Apps can also be classified under five different categories based on their utility: (a) lifestyle mobile apps, (b) social media apps, (c) pre-installed apps, (d) entertainment apps and (e) productivity based apps. Lifestyle mobile apps facilitate the lifestyle of an individual. Apps designed for fitness and ordering food can be quoted as examples for a lifestyle-based app. Social media apps are designed for a social purpose. Pre-installed apps, on the other hand, are pre-installed on the mobile. Various options such as calculator, alarm and calendar available on a mobile are considered to be the examples for this category. While the entertainment apps, as the name suggests, are developed with the motive of providing entertainment. Productivity based apps are gaining popularity over the years. These apps enable its users to accomplish a task easily and efficiently. The wallet/pay apps can be quoted as an example of a productivity-based app.

The utility of apps in health care has helped professionals to conserve time and has enabled easy access. Some of the most commonly used apps in information and time management include apps like Evernote and Notability. Information management refers to the storage, updation and sharing of the information. The cloud-based storage and dropbox are some of the most common utilities in information management. The advantage of these utilities is that this storage system is dynamic, that is, information stored on one system can be accessed through any other system also. These utilities need not be downloaded from the app store and are available as pre-loaded apps on many phones. Time management apps are used to schedule appointments and meetings. The EPIC system in collaboration with Apple Inc has developed an app called Epic which would enable easy access to its users. Team Viewer is yet another app which helps in easy access.

Later the apps extended into other areas of health care like clinical decision making and training. Diagnosaurus is one of the most commonly used app in decision making. The details of a client regarding the symptoms, signs and tests administered can be entered on the app where the possible diagnosis and the other conditions with overlapping symptoms can be seen. The client can use the app to get a condition diagnosed or to obtain a second opinion. Apps are being considerably used in the field of communication disorders.

A study by Sidock (2011) aimed at evaluating the effectiveness of existing literature that used apps in iOS platform, when delivering speech-language therapy. Whereas, the study provides insight specific to the effectiveness of technology, using search engines such as Google Scholar, PubMed and PsycINFO. Along with this, the researcher used specific key terms such as iPad, speech-language therapy, augmentative communication and so on, for the purpose of searching the appropriate and relevant literature in these lines. A major finding of the study yielded positive results when using iDevices (apps), compared to traditional tools in the treatment of young children. Subsequently, the study stated that it is important that the professional can decide the relevance of the app based on the client's need. The studies, which have yielded positive results when delivering therapy using apps, should be interpreted with caution as they are the preliminary findings.

This needs to be strengthened by conducting more research in the same lines. In a sum, it is important to adopt a holistic approach in treating communication disorders. In other words, traditional therapy and app-based therapy should be clubbed in creating a conducive environment for learning. However, there is a gap in the current scenario as the former and the latter are used separately.

The first literature on the utility of apps in communication disorders was published by Gosnell (2011). Gosnell opines that the utility of the app would maximize the diagnostic and therapeutic power of the clinicians and also it may aid in developing the knowledge of a novice clinician. At the same time, the clinicians should be aware of the fact that no single tool fits all the clients. The apps chosen may be effective for some clients; for others, it may not be as effective. So, the clinician employing app should be sensitive about these facts.

A study by Shane and Costello (1994) on similar lines opined that the clinicians should control the technology and the technology should not control the clinicians. The clinician should understand the purpose of an app. The clinician should also be aware of the limitations of an app. In other words, one single app may not have all the features or utilities required by the clients. The clinician should also have the ability to identify the apps which would serve the clients' need effectively and check if a client would be able to use the app in his/her absence as in-home training. Hence, the apps should be carefully used.

A study by Benedon (2018) aimed at evaluating the attitudes of a certified SLP, in using app-based intervention, through a survey method. In this study, the attitude is assessed by using 48 questions, the researcher yielded positive attitude in 82 per cent SLPs who used app-based speech-language therapy and showed a positive attitude towards the utility of apps in speech-language therapy.

Apps for Articulation Disorders

The term articulation refers to pronunciation. It is described as the production of speech sounds through the organs meant for production (articulators). Difficulty in articulating specific sounds is termed as articulation disorder. The terms misarticulation and speech sound disorder are the synonyms for articulation disorder. According to a study by Fernandez (2009), 50 per cent of the therapists in the US prefer to use apps. Most of the therapists, who use apps, use it the most for treating misarticulation. It accounts for 80 per cent of the total usage. Some of the therapists (12% of the total) used the apps for assessments too. Most of the apps had features to evaluate articulation skills, to determine the pattern of speech sound errors, to consider goals for the therapy, to initiate the therapy and to measure the progress. An app by name 'Speech Trainer 3D' (Smarty Ears LLC 2011; Fernandes 2010) is commonly used for articulation therapy and is available in English. This app can be used for the therapy of the children above four years. The app works on the line: Correct placement is essential for progress. The app has a list of sounds and the therapist should choose the sounds based on the errors produced by the child (considered for therapy). Phonetic placement approach was used for intervention. Once the sound is produced at the level of isolation, the therapist can target the same sound at the level of words, phrases and sentences. However, there are some of the advantages of using these apps over the other, for instance, the apps try to incorporate the most efficient technique in treating articulation disorder, that is, phonetic placement tries to incorporate the sounds across various levels and it also aids in providing visual feedback for each of the sounds based on their production. On the other hand, these apps could not account or teach the hypo/hypernasal speech and are not able to teach compensatory articulation due to constraints of the design employed.

Smarty Speech is the other app which is commonly used for speech therapy. Smarty Speech provides attractive flashcards and has three modules on the place of articulation, manner of articulation and phonological processes. In addition to this, the app has a provision of recording and charting the progress. Smarty Speech is exclusively available for iPhones and is not available on android platforms. The app is available in two versions: a basic version which can be downloaded for free and an advance paid version. Some of the other apps used in articulation therapy include Articulation Station Pro. It is an app where the features are basic and are available in in-game version.

The other equivalents for this app are Webber Photo Articulation and Phonics Studio. ArtikPix (Sailers 2013) is a full-fledged free app available on the iPhone platform in English.

The sounds can be worked in isolation or at the word level. The individual sound level is called decks. The deck can be combined bearing the phonotactic rules. The commonalities between these apps are that the sounds can be worked at isolation, the same sounds can be targeted at the word level, flashcards are provided to target the sounds at the word level, multiple attempts can be made to produce different sounds and successful and failed attempts are denoted by visual feedback. The provision of recording is available in most of these apps. The app is found to be advantageous as it is cost effective and has wide variety of tasks/levels moving from isolation-word level. It also provides feedback for individual who have speech sound disorder. On the other hand, this app is not standardized, doesn't have the opportunity to work on sentence-level error, and not able to track the type of error exhibited, i.e., compensatory, substitution or addition errors. Articulation Station Pro (Hanks and Hanks 2007) allows participants to practice at word, sentence and story level. However, there are 22 phonograms, targeting initial, medial and final position. Where each phonogram has 60 target words respectively. Along with this, provision of recording the performances and a gradation level of movement of tasks is also available. Apparently, there are some advantages of using these apps: training is possible from isolation-word-sentence level along with the gradation of difficulty levels and visual feedback is provided. However, there are some disadvantages of these apps like even though the app can be downloaded free of cost, to update the version and to avail all levels of stimulus it needs to be paid. Also, it is not the standardized app which can be used in articulation intervention.

A review study was carried out by Furlong et al. (2018) where the apps available for speech therapy were reviewed. PRISMA (Preferred Reporting Items for Systematic Reviews and Meta-Analyses) guidelines were used for reviewing. The primary purpose of the study was to find the efficacy of the apps. A systematic search was carried out by the researchers on Google Play and iTunes for 10 months. The search items were accessed through 12 key terms. A total of 5076 apps were identified initially and 132 apps which were unique in terms of operation were reviewed in the second phase. The apps were reviewed in terms of customer feedback, features, resolution, cost etc. In terms of customer feedback, it was noticed that some of the apps were rated high by the users and this did not correlate with the quality of the app and its features. The apps were sequenced in terms of app titles, relevance and popularity. The key terms used to search mattered for the app to be listed. Several duplicates were available for a single app. The apps had many overlapping features. The users preferred low-cost apps over high-cost apps. Free apps were downloaded more compared to priced apps. The cost of the apps did not vary as a function of the features provided and the depth of the topic covered in the apps. More apps were available in Google store compared to the apps available in I store. Hence, the authors concluded that the therapeutic benefit was the main feature on the basis of which the apps were downloaded. The preferences for apps were individualistic and the users downloaded and used the app if they found it useful. Thus, it was difficult to earmark apps based on efficacy. The apps can also be reviewed on the basis of the communication disorder.

Apps for Voice Disorders

Voice refers to laryngeal manipulation of the pulmonary air stream. Pitch, loudness and quality are the different parameters of voice. Voice disorders can be diagnosed by an SPL. However, the diagnosis should be correlated with the signs, symptoms and visualization of the vocal folds. The basic parameters, pitch, loudness and quality are targeted in the apps. Most of the apps can be used by the people of all age ranges including children. The apps meant for voice therapy are meant to provide feedback to the user. This feedback would cover the basic parameters. Voice Analyst (Brady and Brady 2011), developed by Speechtools Ltd, is a popular app for voice therapy in English language. It is available only for iPhones. It provides visual feedback to the user. The app has a provision for the user to mention his/her basic details in terms of age, gender etc. The user can use the sustained phonation app available or can produce the words. The optimum loudness is indicated in the bar and the loudness that a user manages to produce is indicated in the form of a line. Based on whether the line converges with the target bar, goes above or goes below, a participant can modulate the voice. It is especially useful for persons with parkinsonism or dysphonia. It is a paid app. However, there are certain advantages of this app. For instance, it can be used in professional voice therapy to fix the pitch, intensity range and to monitor maximum phonation duration of a client with a voice disorder. Albeit, these type of apps need professional help to explore the items. VoiceMeter Pro (Edtech Monster Limited 2018) also works in the same lines as Voice Analyst. It is available in English. As the apps work based on visual feedback, it may cater to the need of children for whom feedback is essential.

Apps for Fluency Disorders

Fluency refers to the uninterrupted flow of speech at an appropriate rate of speech. Continuity, rate of speech and efforts are the important parameters of fluency. Stuttering, neurogenic stuttering and cluttering are considered as disorders of fluency. Stuttering is the most common disorder of fluency in terms of prevalence. Stuttering can be seen in children as well as adults. The categorization of free and paid apps holds good for stuttering. Speech4Good (McDermott 2013), developed by Balbus company, was one of the earliest app used in stuttering therapy. It works on the principle of delayed auditory feedback (DAF). The DAF provides more processing time, this, in turn, would decrease the dysfluencies as the thought and speech is found to synchronise. Live voice recording is anchored by the software and presented to the person utilising it after a lag of 20–300 milliseconds. The duration can be moderated by the clinician based on clinical judgment. One more app termed as DAF assistant also has the same utility as Speech4Good app. DAF assistant is compatible with iOS as well as Android and is one of the most commonly downloaded app in stuttering management. The feedback can be delayed for the duration of 20–250 milliseconds. In addition to this, the feedback can be varied by shifting the frequency by +/-1 Octave. These apps particularly provide feedback to monitor the rate of speech and are regarded as user-friendly apps; the client can himself fix the target and work on his/her rate of speech. However, the fixation of duration is subjected to variability and requires the client to seek help from professionals. Also, this app doesn't target other kinds of dysfluency such as blocks and repetition.

The rate of speech could be high in persons with stuttering as persons with stuttering rush to finish the content at a rapid rate. 'Metronome pacing' is one of the most preliminary approaches in regulating the rate of speech in persons with stuttering. Speech Pacer (SLP Tap Apps 2013) is an app which can be used for the same purpose. Speech Pacer shows the patient a text to read and moves a text-highlighting cursor along with to pace a user's reading rate. Patient speaks each word, phrase or sentence, as it is highlighted. However, there are various advantages of this app, it aids the patients to slow down the speech by pointing the approximate cursor towards the targeted word. Also, it has the provision of varying the rate based on the present level of the client. On the other hand, this is not user-friendly, he/she requires assistance by a qualified professional. Cool Speech (ByteCool software 2001) is an Android app which can be used for altering the rate of speech in English language. Cool Speech app is available for Android platforms. It was developed with the premise of helping persons with stuttering in establishing self-control. On the other hand, these apps help to regulate the dysfluency using the principle of self-control and give more emphasis on self-feedback.

SpeakMore is an another app used in stuttering therapy. The app has several modules; the first module can be used to assess for stuttering severity. The app has three levels as well: patient, server and the therapist. The patient is supposed to record his speech and save it on the server and the clinician would listen to these samples. In addition to this, the patient would analyse the anxiety on a day-to-day basis and report. The clinician would cross-check it and provide strategies to cope with the problem.

Stuttering Helper (Janus Development Group 2012) is available in English, German, Northern Sami and Spanish languages; it is one more app which can be used for fluency issues. The app gives tips to the persons with stuttering on how to cope with dysfluencies including the tips and strategies to be followed during the moments of stuttering. This app is available on Android and iOS platforms. The app is also available in a software version. The developers of the app claim that the app is not an equivalent of therapy but is to reduce the fear in the mind of persons with stuttering regarding the communication breakdown which is vulnerable in them. Thus, these apps have a vital role in delivering strategies to cope with stuttering. Also, they enable the use of some of the tailored-made situations and practices. FluencyCoach (Janus Development Group 2009) is a popular app available for persons with fluency disorders in English language. The app can be used for the reduction of dysfluencies. Some preloaded samples are available on the app, the person with stuttering is expected to read the same lines in the chorus. The person with stuttering reads the same content displayed simultaneously on the mobile screen. The app is available for download on iOS and Android platforms. 'Choral reading' is one of the main techniques and evidence-based approach in fluency intervention. It is assumed to be a fluency-provoking condition. The chorus can be eventually faded off and the person should be capable of speaking fluently even without a chorus. Thus, this app trains in the fluency skills using normal samples as references. The disordered speech is compared with the reference and this in-turn gives feedback for the participants. However, the app incorporates only choral reading and it is difficult for a patient to generalize in other tasks such as narration and conversation.

Fluency SIS (Smart Intervention Strategies) is one more popular paid app available on iOS platform. The app is used for practice and can be used by a person with stuttering for at-home training. The client can avail therapy and use this app as an adjunct to therapy. The app is available in English. The app has four modules: the first module is to practice gentle onset and the person can rehearse the words until he/she is capable of establishing gentle onset. The second module is for appropriate pausing and phrasing. The pause is assumed to be inappropriate in persons with stuttering. The clients are asked to speak slowly in smaller phrases and sentences initially; gradually, the length and complexity of utterances are increased. The third module indulges the participant in question and answer sessions. Answering to questions in real-time is one of the most difficult aspect seen in persons with stuttering. The fourth module enables its users to rehearse the presentation. This feature enables persons with stuttering to be more confident while confronting situations confidently. Some of the apps are developed with the premise of reducing the anxiety and depression type of factors associated with stuttering.

Apps for Language Disorders

Language is defined as a system of arbitrary vocal symbols, which has shared meaning, used by a group of people for communication. The term 'spoken language disorder' is used to depict language disorders in children; it is a complex phenomenon as it exists with a variety of comorbid conditions like hearing loss and intellectual disability. The therapist must consider these conditions during the process of intervention. Many apps can be used for language intervention in children. More apps are available for language intervention in children compared to any other disorders.

Most of the apps are used to access the materials, flashcards etc. required for therapy. Language Builder is one of the most commonly used apps to treat receptive and expressive language disorder. This app has several modules such as tense builder, prepositions builder and sentence builder. The clinician can opt for the modules based on the ability of the child.

There are some specific apps for vocabulary developing. Language Empire (Simms 2019), Proloquo2Go, Pictello, Splingo's Language Universe are few apps meant for this purpose. iName is a popular app used for both vocabulary building as well as word retrieval difficulties. The app Social Quest (Fernandes 2012) is a special app developed by smarty ears for the intervention of pragmatics used in English language. It is a unique app as it targets pragmatics, unlike the other apps which work on the form and content aspects of the language. Several apps are available on Android platform too. Most of these apps have overlapping features. This app has several merits to its credit for instance; it encompasses all components essential for language learning such as vocabulary building and asking wh-questions. However, on the other hand, it doesn't have the flexibility to add some of the stories pertaining to client interest.

Some of the apps can be used for spoken language disorders secondary to hearing loss. Listen and Speak is one unique app. It has activities targeting detection, discrimination, activities in par with the auditory training aspects considered in the intervention of spoken language disorder with hearing loss.

Alternative and Augmentative Communication (AAC)

It is one of the most established concepts used in therapy. It refers to methods of communication which can replace or substitute the existing form of communication. Two unique apps were developed through Sc@ut Project (Rodríguez-Fórtiz et al. 2009, 1348–1352) and Picaa (Fernandez 2009, 423–432). The common feature between the two apps is that both these apps use communication boards for communication. The basic module has pictures, which can be used by patients for immediate communication. The second module has letters which can be clubbed for forming words. The other modules have symbols which can be used by patients or their caregivers. Some of the most common AAC apps are summarised in Table 3.1.

Table 3.1 *List of Alternative and Augmentative Communication Apps*

Lingraphica (Medical Technology Limited 1990, New Jersey)	A communication device for aphasia with a vocabulary of pictures that talk in a natural human voice
PEAT TM	Patented automatic planning features include floating tasks and scripts
Gus Talking Keyboard (AssistiveWare, 2015, Washington)	A text-to-speech program that combines an on-screen keyboard with an exceptionally clear synthetic voice
Gus Multimedia Speech System (AssistiveWare, 2015, Washington)	Unlimited number of pages of pre-programmed words and phrases
Windbag-3 (Augmentative communication consultants 1999)	Text-based communication aid program. Messages may be in the synthetic or digitized speech.

Grid-2 (Smartbox Assistive Technology 2006)	Communication aid, using symbols or text to build sentences
SpeechPRO (Speech Technology Centre Limited 1990)	Includes an alphabetic vocabulary file named wordlist
ClozePro (Inclusive Technology 2001)	Used for Reading, comprehension and vocabulary skills
Clicker 5 (Crick Software 2005)	Includes write with whole words, phrases or pictures

Apps for Children with Autism

A variety of apps are available for children with autism, iPrompts is an app which is popularly used in children with autism. It can be used by caregivers and patients for scheduling. The app provides a visual support tool to enhance communication. A complex activity can be divided into simple steps and can be accomplished sequentially. The app Chorewars is also meant for the same purpose. The app Social Express provides a variety of communication situations, where persons with autism can rehearse communication situations in advance so that communication breakdown can be prevented. Everybody Happy is another app which can be used for the same purpose. Calm Counter and Calm Myself Down are some of the apps to prevent the anxiety arising from a communication breakdown. Many apps are also available for persons with a learning disability. ModMath is a free app which can be used in tackling reading and writing problems. It also has a module on maths for children exhibiting problems in maths. Dyslexia Toolbox also serves the same purpose.

Aphasia

Several apps are available for persons with aphasia also. Aphasia refers to acquired language disorder secondary to acquired conditions such as stroke, trauma and tumour. Constant Therapy (CT) is one of the most popular apps available for aphasia. It was developed at Boston University and is adapted to Indian context (Goswami, Kiran and Radhakrishna 2018). It has modules like calendar tasks, categories, feature tasks, letter to phoneme tasks and map tasks. However, these apps are custom made and necessary changes could be made according to the clients' needs. These apps need good upper motor skills to perform the tasks with ease. Also, this does not incorporate eye gaze technique in general.

A study by Hoge (2014) was conducted with the aim to conclude how SLPs in medical set-up choose between the app-based intervention and traditional intervention-based approach. This study incorporated a survey method to take the opinion of SLPs, about using app-based intervention in a medical set-up. Results of the study showed that over 82 per cent SLPs who work in medical set up use app-based intervention and feel comfortable while delivering this approach to persons with aphasia.

A study by Stark and Warburton (2018) was carried out to investigate the effectiveness of self-delivered therapy in persons with chronic aphasia. Some of the apps were provided to persons with aphasia and they were asked to use these apps on their own. Result of the study indicated, that there was an increasing trend in response to post-treatment assessment in chronic expressive aphasia. From this study, we can infer that self-delivered therapy via an app is beneficial.

Lingraphica is a set of dedicated communication devices for adults with aphasia. It is available in a laptop model and an app version. The app version can be used for functional communication as well as for promoting verbal mode of communication in persons with aphasia. The AllTalk is a lightweight, ultra-sleek laptop which works on the basis of eye gaze technique and is designed to help even to the persons with severe aphasia. The primary premise is to prevent communication breakdown in aphasia and to promote functional communication. MiniTalk—a tablet model—is used for improving lifestyle. SmallTalk—a family of free apps—can be used for functional communication. TalkPath Therapy is an app for functional communication. TactusTherapy (Sutton and Carter 2011) is an app similar to CT. It was developed by TactusTherapy Solutions and it is a multi-module app. It has modules on comprehension, naming repetition, reading and writing.

Some of the apps developed for persons with dementia include Schedule it, Daily dairy and daily register. These apps primarily enable persons with dementia to schedule their activity daily so that it would facilitate the activities and reduce the impact on daily living.

CONSIDERATIONS WHILE DOWNLOADING AN APP

The utility of apps with children is subjected to slight controversy as some proponents believe that the mobile apps would lead to more distraction and the utility is limited. DeCurtis and Dawn (2011) have proposed the '7 Ps' to be considered while using these apps.

These '7 Ps' principles are as follows:

1. Preparation: The reason as to why a mobile app should be used along with toys is to be justified.
2. Participants: The probable candidacy has to be decided where the client's age, intelligent quotient, and associated problems should be given weightage while deciding on the apps.
3. Parameters: The clinician or the parent should decide on what all aspects of communication have to be addressed by the app.
4. Purpose: The clinician should know the purpose of using an app and it should co-inside with the goal taken up in therapy.
5. Positioning: Positioning follows the purpose, where the clinician should decide the duration for using the app and the duration to be dedicated to face-to-face therapy.
6. Playtime: Playtime is when the clinician makes the app more friendly to the user (child). The app should be introduced as a part of play so that the child becomes more connected with the app.
7. Potential: The last step is termed as potential which deals in the ability of the clinician to link the activities prescribed on the app with activities of daily living so that the actual purpose of the app is achieved.

The general considerations to be considered by the clinicians while prescribing app include:

1. Understanding of the problem
2. Knowing the extent of the problem
3. Co-morbid conditions

4. Attention abilities
5. The app meets the requirements
6. The cost of the app
7. Judging, if the app would serve the purpose
8. Deciding, if the therapy as a whole is imparted through the app or if the utility of the app is just confined to home training.
9. Tracking the progress after usage
10. Changing the app periodically, if needed
11. Suggesting the patients regarding the modules to be targeted
12. Counselling of the client on the impediments of the apps

The factors to be considered by the patients/caregivers include:

1. Understanding the problem
2. Understanding the purpose of app usage
3. Knowing the limits of the apps
4. The modules to be used
5. Charting progress
6. Taking periodic advice from the clinician
7. Changing the app or stop using it, if the progress is limited

User Perspectives on Apps

The users of the apps such as patients with communication disorders or their caregivers use a particular app based on the following facts:

1. Cost of the app: People prefer free apps over paid apps.
2. Aspects covered: The users may be attracted to the app which encompasses a variety of domains than the app which contains fewer domains.
3. Visual Resolution: The users prefer apps which look attractive and are eye-catching.
4. Provision for recording and receiving suggestions: This factor also would provoke the users in considering apps.

Many apps are available for download. The apps are listed according to their popularity and the number of downloads, the listing of the apps does not suggest that the apps available at the front are more popular. The users must know the name and the features of the apps for better and effective usage.

IMPEDIMENTS OF APPS

Many apps are available for the same purpose. Some of the apps may have common features while few other apps may have special features which are unique. The clinicians should identify the apps based on the features and advice the users regarding them. The purpose of introducing an app should be clearly specified. The efficacy of apps may not be determined or may be difficult in determining owing to diversity, hence, no app is universal. Most of the apps are available in English and not in regional languages, this limits the popularity of the apps. The users of the app should remember that the apps are no replacement for therapy. Hence, the apps should be used carefully.

FUTURE OF THE APPS

The following facts can be incorporated in regards to the utility of apps in communication disorders:

1. Low-cost apps available for download: Some of the apps are costly, this impedes the usage. The development of low-cost apps will solve this problem.
2. Parallel apps on Android and iOS: The iOS has more apps compared to Android and the apps available are also different. Hence, there is a need to draw parallels between the two.
3. Establishing an interface with the clinicians and live discussions may enhance the usage of apps.
4. Efficacy studies should be carried out which may provide more evidence on the utility of an app.

CONCLUSION

The apps are the advent of technology and have revolutionized the field of health care. The utility of apps has been extended to the field of speech-language pathology. Numerous apps have been used by both parents/caregivers of children with speech-language problems as well as the SLPs. Parents may use it to complement therapy and for at-home training while an SLP uses it for various purposes such as stimulus presentation, demonstrating a technique and providing feedback to their clients. An app may have several merits as well as demerits and no app is complete. The usage of an app is warranted to the purpose of usage. There is a dearth of studies determining the efficacy of the apps, thus, limiting their utility. However, apps can be used as an adjunct to speech-language therapy and have all the potential to facilitate the process of therapy.

REFERENCES

Benedon, Tessa Alexandra. 2018. 'Speech-Language Pathologists' Practices and Attitudes Towards App Use in Therapy.' *Theses and Dissertation*. 1748. Available at: https://dc.uwm.edu/etd/1748 (accessed on 19 December 2019).

Brady, Sam, and Garry Brady. 2011. Voice Analyst. Speech Tools Limited. Available at: http.//www.speechtool.com/ (accessed on 19 December 2019).

ByteCool Software Ltd. 2001. *CoolSpeech*. Available at: http://www.bytecool.com/coolspch.htm (accessed on 19 December 2019).

Crick Software. 2005. Clicker 5. Available at: https://www.bltt.org/software/clicker5/ (accessed on 19 December 2019).

DeCurtis, Lisa Luna, and Ferrer Dawn. 2011. 'Toddlers and Technology: Teaching the Techniques.' *The ASHA Leader* 16 (11). https://doi.org/10.1044/leader.FTR5.16112011.np

Edtech Monster limited. 2018. *Voice meter Pro*. Available at: https://apps.apple.com/us/app/voice-meter-pro/id686934049 (accessed on 19 December 2019).

Fernandes, Barbara. 2010. *Smarty Ears*. Available at: https://www.smartyearsapps.com/ (accessed on 19 December 2019).

Fernandes, Barbara. 2012. Smarty Ears. *Social Quest*. Available at: https://apps.apple.com/us/app/social-quest/id556089006 (accessed on 19 December 2019).

Fernandez, Alvaro. 2009. 'Designing and Supporting Cooperative and Ubiquitous Learning Systems for People with Special Needs.' *OTM Workshop*, 423–432. Berlin: Springer.

Furlong, Lisa, Morris Meg, Tanya Serry, and Shane Erickson. (2018). 'Mobile apps for treatment of speech.' *PLoS One*, 13 (8). Available at: https://doi.org/10.1371/journal.pone.0201513 (accessed on 19 December 2019).

Gosnell, Jessica. 2011. 'How to Conduct a Clinical Feature Matching Process.' *11th Annual Conference on Augmentative and Alternative Communication*, Orlando, FL.

Goswami Satyapal, Swati Kiran, and Vimala Radhakrishna. 2018. 'Adaptation of Constant Therapy to Kannada and Hindi.' *AIISH Research Funded Project*, Mysuru (Unpublished).

Hanks, Heidi, and Chris Hanks. 2007. *Little Bee Speech*. Articulation Station. Available at: http://littlebeespeech.com/articulation_station.php (accessed on 19 December 2019).

Hoge, Taryn Louise. 2014. 'Speech-Language Pathologists' Use of iPad Technologies for Persons with Aphasia.' Doctoral Dissertation, Wichita State University, Wichita, KS, USA.

Inclusive Technology. 2001. *ClozePro*. Available at: http://www.inclusive.co.uk/clozepro-p2168# (accessed on 19 December 2019).

Janus Development Group. 2009. *Fluency Coach*. Available at: https://www.fluencycoach.com/ (accessed on 19 December 2019). NC: Greenville.

Janus Development Group. 2012. *Stuttering Helper*. Available at: https://apps.apple.com/us/app/stuttering-helper/id578182856 (accessed on 19 December 2019).

McDermott, Jack. 2013. *Speech4Good*. Balbus Speech. Available at: https://www.mnsu.edu/comdis/kuster/appsforstuttering.html (accessed on 19 December 2019).

Medical Technology Ltd. 1990. *Lingraphica*. Available at: https://www.aphasia.com/ (accessed on 19 December 2019).

McKinnon, David H., McLeod Sharynne, and Reilly Sheena. 2007. 'The Prevalence of Stuttering, Voice, and Speech-Sound Disorders in Primary School Students in Australia.' *Language, Speech, and Hearing Services in Schools* 38 (January): 05–15.

Owens, Robert E. 2006. 'Development of Communication, Language, and Speech.' *Human Communication Disorders: An Introduction*. 7th ed. Boston, MA: Pearson/Allyn & Bacon.

Rodríguez-Fórtiz, M. J., J. L. González, A. Fernández, M. Entrena, M. J. Hornos, A. Pérez, A. Carrillo, and L. Barragán. 2009. 'Sc@ut: Developing Adapted Communicators for Special Education.' *Procedia—Social and Behavioural Sciences*, 1 (1), 1348–1352.

Sailers, Eric. 2013. *Artikpix*. Available at: https://apps.apple.com/us/app/artikpix-full/id356720379 (accessed on 19 December 2019).

Sidock, J. 2011. 'Critical Review: Is the Integration of Mobile Device Apps' into Speech and Language Therapy Effective Clinical Practice.' School of Communication Sciences and Disorders, University of Western Ontario.

Shane, Howard C., and John M. Costello. 1994. *Augmentative Communication Assessment and the Featurematching Process*. Annual Convention of the American Speech Language Hearing Association, New Orleans, LA, USA.

Simms, Rosie. 2019. *Language Empires*. Smarty Ears LLC. Available at: https://apps.apple.com/us/app/languageempires/id562910097 (accessed on 19 December 2019).

SLP Tap Apps. 2013. *Speech Pacer and SLP Dysfluency Plus*. Available at: http://www.slp-tapappa.com/slp-tapapps.com (accessed on 15 August 2013).

Smartbox Assistive Technology. 2006. *Grid 2*. Available at: https://thinksmartbox. com/download-the-grid-2/ (accessed on 19 December 2019).

Speech Technology Centre Limited. 1990. *SpeechPro*. Available at: https://speech-pro.com/ (accessed on 19 December 2019).

Stark, Brielle C., and Elizabeth A. Warburton. 2018. 'Improved Language in Chronic Aphasia after Self-delivered iPad Speech Therapy.' *Neuropsychological Rehabilitation*, 28 (5), 818–831.

Sutton, Megan, and Ben Carter. 2011. *Tactus Therapy*. Canada. Available at: https:// tactustherapy.com (accessed on 19 December 2019).

Telerehabilitation in Stuttering

Rakesh C. V. and Santosh Maruthy

INTRODUCTION

Stuttering is a fluency disorder that affects the communication abilities of an individual in a social context. Stuttering comprises both overt (repetitions, blocks, and prolongations) and covert behaviours (anxiety, shame, fear and negative attitude). Typically stuttering begins in early childhood, that is, between the age of two and five years (Guitar 2013; Ratner and Silverman 2000; Yairi, Ambrose and Grinager 2005), and is prevalent in both children and adults (Hull et al. 1976). Spontaneous recovery in young children without any treatment is considered to be one of the most noteworthy features of stuttering (Yairi and Seery 2015). A varied range of spontaneous recovery rates has been reported in the literature, which ranges from 23 per cent to 80 per cent (Craig et al. 2002). Although a large number of children recover from stuttering without any formal treatment, a substantial number of children fail to do so.

The quality of life of a person who stutters (PWS) may be affected due to the existence of overt (interruption to the smooth flow of speech) and covert stuttering behaviours. Studies have reported that children who stutter (CWS) develop more negative speech associated attitude (Guttormsen, Kefalianos and Næss 2015) and negative quality of mood (Johnson et al. 2010) when compared to their fluent speaking peer groups. The negative effects of stuttering have been reported to start during preschool age and aggravate during adolescence (Guttormsen, Kefalianos and Næss 2015; Iverach et al. 2016). Stuttering related anxiety is one of the common problems identified in both children and adults (Iverach et al. 2016). Persistence of stuttering not only hampers the speaking abilities of the individual, but also it exposes the PWS at higher risk of developing psychological problems.

To minimize these negative effects, early identification and treatment of stuttering are essential as the success rate in CWS is greater (>90%) when compared to adults who stutter (AWS) (50%–70%) (Onslow, Andrews and Lincoln 1994). Further, the CWS take lesser treatment duration with lower relapse rate (0%) when compared to AWS (50%) (Franken 1987). Disfluencies can be reduced or eliminated with early identification and evidence-based intervention programmes for stuttering, which involves intense and prolonged face-to-face contact with the speech-language pathologist (SLP). In adults, the maintenance and generalization of therapy gains can be difficult or challenging (Theodoros 2008). These aspects of an intervention programme can be challenging to access for the patients who reside in remote locations and for those who face transportation issues, financial issues and patients who cannot access the services due to mobility reasons (Theodoros 2008; Wilson, Onslow and Lincoln 2004). This may also be due to the accumulation of SLP's in urban areas (Carey et al. 2010; Kully 2002). Telepractice could be a connecting bridge between the SLPs, who are experienced in delivering evidence-based practice and the patients who require the treatment against all the odds mentioned above.

TREATMENT PROTOCOLS FOR STUTTERING

Numerous intervention programmes currently exist for PWS. The present chapter contains three primary intervention programmes that are delivered through telepractice: (a) Lidcombe programme, (b) Camperdown programme, and (c) an integrative approach, which includes a combination of widely-accepted stuttering treatments (e.g., avoidance reduction, stuttering modification and fluency shaping).

One of the established evidence-based parent-delivered intervention programmes for CWS is the Lidcombe programme (Jones et al. 2005). In this programme, the parents/caregivers are taught to deliver verbal contingencies in response to their child's speech. Self-evaluation, acknowledgement and praise are the contingencies used for stutter-free speech; request for self-correction and acknowledgement are used for unambiguous stutters (Wilson et al., 2004). Even though it is very popular and effective in treating CWS, except for one study which is still under trial phase (Koushik, Shenker and Onslow 2009), there are no evidence or attempts made to utilize this successful programme in adults or school-aged population.

In general, adults having persistent stuttering are less reactive to treatment (Guitar 2013). Besides, adults who stutter generally develop negative speech associated attitude, social maladjustments, reduced performance at workplace and phobias (Carey et al. 2010). Currently, persistent stuttering is treated using the speech-restructuring technique, in which the speech is altered at the level of articulation, phonation and breathing (Carey et al. 2010). Speech-restructuring generally involves prolonged speech such as Camperdown programme (Carey et al. 2010; O'Brian, Packman and Onslow 2008). In the Camperdown programme, the participant will be provided with spoken models of prolonged speech and the participants are free to use any features of the speech which will enable them to speak fluently and more comfortably (O'Brian, Packman and Onslow 2008). The last treatment approach is the integrated treatment approach, which includes evidenced-based protocols like avoidance reduction, stuttering modification, desensitization and fluency shaping (Kully 2000).

TELEPRACTICE AND STUTTERING

Telerehabilitation is the process of delivering health care services to the patients through dedicated site-based videoconferencing, telephone and personal computer-based videoconferencing (Skype), where distance is the critical factor.

Telehealth services can be high-tech or low-tech depending upon the medium employed. Generally, the high-tech includes dedicated site-based videoconferencing and the low-tech comprises telephonic communication and emails. Since the last two decades, with the advancement of communication technology, tele-assessment and treatment of children and adults who stutter has gained popularity due to its ease of accessibility, time and cost-effectiveness. Telehealth services may be delivered through one or more of the following channels; (a) synchronous treatment consists of dedicated site-based videoconferencing/personal computer-based videoconferencing (Skype), (b) telephone-based intervention, (c) asynchronous treatment consisting of pre-recorded videos, messages and emails and (d) hybrid, which is a combination of direct (traditional therapy) and telehealth services (Cherney and Van Vuuren 2012).

Synchronous treatment mode encompasses of live videoconferencing where the SLP delivers the treatment online in real-time and the treatment programme is client-directed. Counselling and treatment plans are hand-tailored based on the signs and symptoms of the patient. Whereas, asynchronous mode consists of emails, which addresses the typical set of signs and symptoms of the problem without addressing individual patients details. The few advantages of this modality are, it is fast, easy to use and its privacy (with end to end encryption) followed by uncertainty regarding the usage of traditional counselling (Efstathiou 2009).

However, the preferred channel for delivering telehealth services for the treatment of stuttering is dedicated site-based videoconferencing/personal computer-based videoconferencing (Skype) because it helps in building client-clinician rapport which is very close to direct method of intervention (Richards and Viganó 2013). Also, the comparison studies between synchronous and asynchronous delivery mode have reported that there is an increased anxiety level in the clients in asynchronous mode due to the presence of time delay (Richards and Viganó 2013). Lastly, considering the nature of stuttering disorder like occasional inaudible pauses and physical concomitants, the video-based synchronous delivery mode will increase the accuracy of the service delivery; especially when it involves the assessment.

Telehealth services delivery model is effective in treating speech and language disorders (Theodoros 2008). Stuttering intervention via telemode is more feasible and has potentials for good prognosis because usually, the gains that are made within the clinic situations are not generalized to other situations (O'Brian, Packman and Onslow 2008). If effectively implemented telehealth services delivery model has the potential to enhance the intervention programme gains and to reduce some of the barriers to traditional face-to-face therapy such as distance and cost.

Last two decades have witnessed a considerable amount of research and clinical activity about telerehabilitation in stuttering. Studies have been conducted in a sequence of trials, with most of them being in Phase I followed by few studies in the Phase II trial stages. The present chapter aims to evaluate and investigate the telehealth practices and research in PWS to date. The chapter consists of a qualitative review of articles and provides a brief introduction to stuttering intervention programmes, which are adapted and delivered through telehealth practices and summarize the evidence for the same when delivered through telemode.

METHOD FOR LITERATURE SEARCH AND SELECTION OF THE STUDIES

The studies, which are included in this chapter, were chosen from a systematic electronic search of the literature in Research Gate, PubMed, Google Scholar and J-gate. Also, the back-reference manual search was carried out. The search was restricted to peer-reviewed journals and original articles, which were written in English. All the studies included were related to telerehabilitation of stuttering. Telerehabilitation here includes webcam or videoconferencing therapy, emails and telephonic conversations. The study designs that are included here are Phase I and Phase II studies and randomized control studies. All the studies had PWS as participants categorized into children, adolescents and adults. Conclusively, a total of 15 studies available online up to December 2018, were considered. Shortlisted studies were analysed in terms of the following major characteristics: (a) intervention programmes, (b) outcome measures and (c) research designs.

The method followed for literature search and selection of the studies are depicted in Figure 4.1.

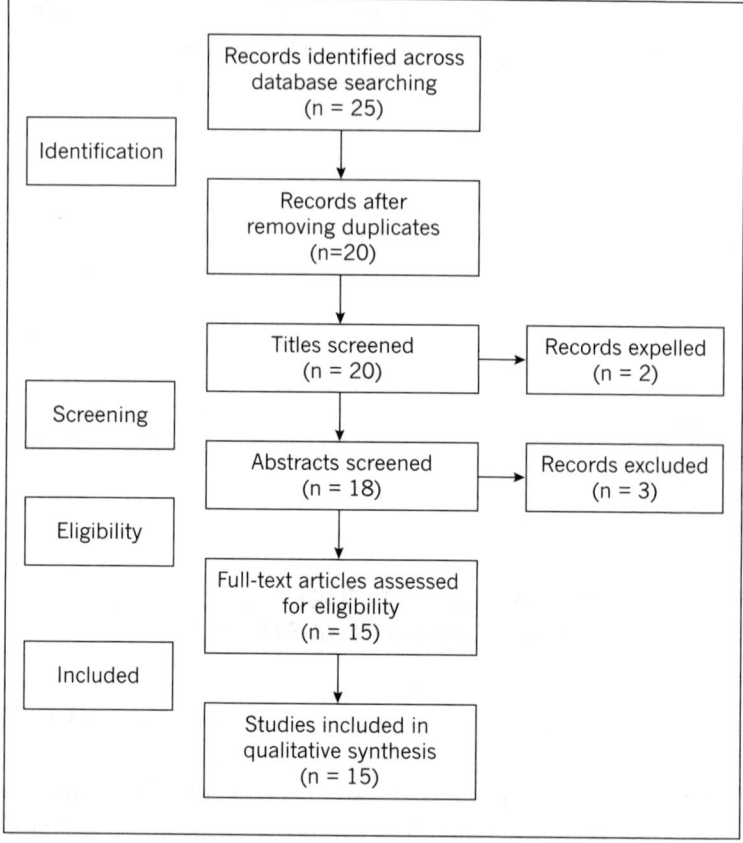

Figure 4.1 *The Preferred Reporting Items for Systematic Review and Meta-Analyses (PRISMA) Flowchart Outlining the Steps Followed in This Chapter*

INTERVENTION PROGRAMMES FOR THE PERSONS WHO STUTTER

There were several programmes available in the literature that helps in treating stuttering. The Lidcombe and Camperdown programmes are two such programmes that are widely used for treating stuttering. These programmes have been modified and delivered through tele-mode and are found to be effective in reducing disfluencies. Studies have been conducted using Phase I, Phase II and Randomized Clinical Trials (RCTs). The details of the mentioned programmes are explained in the section below.

Lidcombe Programme

Lidcombe programme is a behavioural treatment targeting children's stuttered speech (Onslow et al. 2017). It is a parent-implemented programme based on the principles of operant conditioning. Here the children are not instructed to change their customary speech pattern in any way. Parents do not alter speech and language habits or the family lifestyle in any way. Parents only deliver verbal contingencies for fluent and stuttered speech separately. The measurement includes the severity rating scales (SRs) within and outside the clinic situations. SRs provide parents and/or clinicians a way to plan the presentation of the verbal contingencies. Here the clinician and the parent decide to plan and target the particular occasions defined by a degree of stuttering to provide verbal contingency. The measurements also include per cent syllables stuttered (%SS) at the initial visit to the clinic. It is measured during a conversation where the child displays stuttering. The verbal contingencies used in the Lidcombe programme are grossly divided into two groups: verbal contingencies for stutter-free speech and verbal contingencies for moments of unambiguous stuttering. The verbal contingencies for stutter-free speech include praise, request for self-evaluation and acknowledgement. The verbal contingencies for moments of unambiguous stuttering include acknowledgement and request for self-correction.

The Lidcombe programme consists of two stages. The goal during the Stage I of the treatment is no stuttering/almost no stuttering; Stage II aims at no stuttering or almost no stuttering to be sustained for a long time and also to maintain the absence or low level of stuttering attained compared to the previous stage. It is reported that most of the children with some fleeting signs of stuttering with a mean age of 5 years, after they began Stage I, have chances of relapse after successful Lidcombe programme treatment. The stages incorporated in the programme are described below.

Stage I clinic visits: Stage I requires the parent/caregiver, along with the child, to visit the clinician once each week. During the visit, the following sequence is followed: (a) child's conversation, where, after a conversation with the child, the clinician measures the stuttering severity rating, as well as the percentage of syllables stuttered. After which the clinician (b) checks for the parent severity rating, based on the rating and then (c) a discussion concerning the progress of the child during the previous week is done, where, details on the sessions planned, frequency and type of verbal contingencies used are discussed. After which the (d) parents demonstrate verbal contingencies used and the clinician monitors the session. Following which, the (e) clinician discusses the verbal contingencies demonstrated by the parent and suggests the required modifications, if any. Subsequent to this, (f) the parent and clinician plan and the clinician demonstrates to the parent any changes in the treatment procedures for the following week, and (g) the session is concluded by summarizing the treatment for the following week.

Stage II clinic visits: The Stage II visits would be for 30 minutes. Here the number of verbal contingencies that have been used during natural conversations since the last visit are discussed. In cases where the child has successfully met the goals, the clinician progresses to the next step. In cases where the child is unable to meet the required goals, progress to the next step is not recommended. In such instances, the clinician either (a) schedules an appointment for the next week and makes recommendations regarding management for the child's increased stuttering, (b) schedules a return to an earlier stage or (c) returns the child to stage II. Stage II is continued until the child can sustain the goals for about a year or so. At the completion of stage II, the parents are counselled to contact the clinician if any relapse occurs.

Adaptation of Lidcombe Programme to Telerehabilitation Mode

The tele-Lidcombe programme is delivered through the synchronous modality only. The telehealth adaptation of the Lidcombe programme is similar to the traditional Lidcombe programme (in accordance to the treatment manual) with few modifications with respect to the mode of delivery of the programme, that is, (a) the mode of delivery is via video teleconferencing/telephone conversation, (b) substituting clinical visits with scheduled telephonic conversations, (c) the speech sample recording for the percentage of syllables stuttered at initial consultation during the clinical visit is replaced by frequent recording in everyday situations by the parents, (d) there is also the availability of hotlines for consultations with the experts, (e) in the televersion of the Lidcombe programme, the real-time recordings are emailed to the clinician or sometimes measured by the trained parent, to add on, the parents are provided with video training materials, (f) the clinician and the parents rate the stuttering severity based on the recorded video samples instead of real-time video samples, (g) during subsequent consultations, the feedback is provided to the parents by the clinician, concerning the implementation of verbal contingencies based on the video samples mailed by the parents and, (h) the contact between the child and the clinician is infrequent in the televersion of the programme as compared to the standard version of the programme.

The Lidcombe programme has been adapted to telemode with the incorporation of the modifications as mentioned earlier (Wilson, Onslow and Lincoln 2004). Few researchers have adapted and studied the usefulness and feasibility of the Lidcombe programme via telemode. The details of the same are given below.

In a case study by Harrison, Wilson and Onslow (1999), a five-year-and-ten-month-old boy who had severe stuttering since four years was treated using an adapted Lidcombe programme through telephone consultations. The whole programme was carried using telephonic consultations and audio and video recordings of the child's speech mailed to the SLP. The per cent SS measured before beginning the programme ranged from 12.4 to 17.7 per cent SS, indicating severe stuttering. The child was found to attain near-zero stuttering levels after almost nine months of treatments with 25 consultations. Per cent SS was reported to have reached 0.1 at 23 months post-treatment measure and syllable per minute increased to 198 from 101 during pre-treatment measure. Thus, the authors postulated that distant delivery mode of the Lidcombe programme through the telephone to be a viable solution for families that have limited access to clinical set-up to receive the standard programme.

Wilson, Onslow and Lincoln (2004) reported the outcome of five children aged between 3.5 years to 5.7 years who received the Lidcombe programme through telephonic consultations for stuttering. In addition to the telephonic consultations, video training materials were mailed to the parents to train them to carry out the programme and provide appropriate contingencies. Per cent SS and SPM were measured from video or audio recordings of the children's speeches. All the children were found to reach the clinical criterion to finish Stage I. At 12 months post-treatment, two children showed 1.0 per cent SS and two showed less than 2.0 per cent SS while one child showed a relapse of stuttering. All the parents except one reported being highly satisfied with the telehealth delivery of the Lidcombe programme. Hence, the authors suggested that distant delivery of the Lidcombe programme would be more efficient if further supplemented with videoconferencing.

A Phase II trial of telehealth delivery of the Lidcombe programme was carried out by Lewis et al. (2008). Out of a total of 22 children recruited for the present study, nine children were randomly assigned to the experimental group and 13 children to control group. The experimental group received the tele-Lidcombe programme through telephonic conversations by an experienced clinician, whereas the control group received no treatment. To carry out a Phase II trial, the total number of responders was calculated from the sample. The responders were defined as the children who show more significant than 80 per cent reduction in per cent SS within nine months post-randomization. With the mean of 49 consultations to complete stage I, six children in experimental and two in the control group have been reported to meet the criteria of responders. The mean per cent SS scores for the experimental and control groups were 1.1 and 1.9 respectively compared to 6.7 and 4.5 for the experimental and control group respectively at the time of randomization. Thus, the authors suggest that this Phase II trial further warrants the need for phase III trial with a higher number of participants randomized. Also, this study augments the evidence of other studies that have reported benefits of teledelivery of Lidcombe programme for participants with limited access to clinical set-up.

The usefulness and feasibility of Phase I treatment of Internet and webcam-based Lidcombe programme was explored by O'Brian, Smith and Onslow (2014), on three preschool children who stuttered. This research was taken up in order to overcome the potential barriers with the standard delivery of Lidcombe programme such as access to clinical set-up every week and problems faced during generalization from clinical to natural settings. Both assessment and treatment were carried out using a webcam and any of the participants or parents did no clinical visit during the treatment. All the three children were diagnosed as having stuttering during a webcam session and pre-treatment stuttering rates were calculated as baselines. Further, before the commencement of treatment, the parents were asked to complete a questionnaire to provide information on family history, developmental history and also about the nature and severity of stuttering perceived. The percentage of syllables stuttered were measured using the audio recordings of the child's speech during play. Two recordings per assessment were done by a researcher through telephone: one at home with a family member and another one away from home with a non-family member. The authors found the children to have less than 1.0 of per cent SS at the end of six months post completion of stage I. To complete stage I of the Lidcombe programme the children took a mean of 34 consultations and 40 weeks. The parent-reported stuttering severity rating at six months post completion of stage I was two (extremely mild stuttering) for one child while the other two parents reported of no stuttering behaviour. The programme has also been shown to yield better parent satisfaction and the parents found a webcam-based Lidcombe programme to be beneficial, comfortable, convenient and cost-effective. Thus, the authors concluded the webcam treatment to be better than the only telephone-based Lidcombe programme for children who have limited access to the clinically-based standard programme.

Bridgman et al. (2016) compared standard clinical and webcam-based Lidcombe programme. Using a randomized control trial method, out of 49 children recruited for the present study, 24 children were assigned to the control group and 25 children to the experimental group. Control group received traditional Lidcombe programme treatment for stuttering, whereas the experimental group received tele-Lidcombe programme delivered through webcam by the same clinician who was blinded during the assessments. Children in the age range of three to five years eleven months, the persistence of stuttering for more than six months, with adequate English language skills were recruited. Per cent SS and number of consultations to complete stage I was measured as primary outcomes.

Further, secondary outcome measures considered included per cent SS at 18 months post-randomization; SR measured by parents and also parents perceived the relationship with the child and clinician. In the control and experimental group, per cent SS and SR were shown to have a significant difference compared to pre-randomization measurement. However, the authors reported insufficient evidence to show differences between standard and webcam-based Lidcombe programme. Besides these insufficiencies, the webcam-based programme has been reported to show similar outcomes of the standard programme. Therefore, authors have found it to be a reliable and efficient programme for treating children with stuttering who have limited access to standard delivery of the Lidcombe programme.

Camperdown Programme

The Camperdown programme was described by O'Brian et al. (2016) as a behavioural treatment that can be best used with adults and adolescents older than 12 years. The severity of stuttering is from mild to severe degree of stuttering to reduce the stuttering during everyday talking. The programme consists of a training mode that can be used to demonstrate and teach speech which can be spoken in a relaxed and exaggerated manner. The programme includes clinical measurement and self-management procedures. The programme addresses social anxiety management and consists of four stages, which include (a) teaching treatment components (b) establishing natural-sounding stutter-free speech with the clinician (c) generalization and (d) maintaining stuttering control.

Stage I: The first stage consists of four to five 45–60 mins consultation. First, the client is given an overview of the programme. This stage includes the client being able to use the speech measures like the 9-point Stuttering Severity Scale and the 9-point Fluency Technique Scale (FTS) and use fluency techniques to understand and learn to regulate their stuttering using the provided training model. At this stage, speech-related anxiety is common for adults; thus, it is essential to have a clinical measure for speech-related anxiety. Subjective Units of Distress Scale (SUDS) is a widely used scale that allows the client to record scores daily for speaking situations used at this stage. The transition from stage I to stage II is when the self-scores on Stuttering Severity Scale of the client resembles that of the clinician's scores and use of the fluency technique is close to the training model and a stuttering severity score of zero. It is also required for clients to report that they are in control of their stuttering to move to the next stage. Further, the client should be able to identify different fluency technique scores from the recordings or when demonstrated by the clinician.

Stage II: The programme uses natural-sounding fluency techniques to control stuttering during everyday talking by shaping the speech. Stage II involves a series of repeated fluency Cycles. During this stage, the clients must be able to (a) consolidate their imitation of the training model fluency technique, (b) work with the clinician to develop an individualized, natural-sounding fluency technique that they find acceptable for stuttering control, (c) practise self-evaluation skills and (d) develop problem-solving skills to assist themselves at a later stage. To move on to the next stage it is required that the clients use the fluency technique during their everyday talking. It is essential that the tailor-made fluency technique, to control stuttering at a conversation level has been developed before the clients move to stage III of the programme.

Stage III: This stage begins when clients are able to converse with the clinician, for the entire session, with the stuttering severity score of 0–1 and an acceptable fluency technique score. Here, it is confirmed that the clients can still use a fluency technique to control their stuttering and are able to compare their speech measures during the consultation with those of the clinician. The clients must be able to revise, review and report their stuttering severity, fluency technique and speech-related anxiety scores from their everyday talking. The clients must also be able to discuss the speech measures, interpret them and plan the required strategies to resolve any related difficulties. The clients must be able to come up with an individualized hierarchy of targeted speaking situations to assist the transfer of their fluency technique into their everyday talking. The clients must also be able to plan, modify and summarize treatment programmes/changes for the upcoming week based on speech measures. The transition from stage III to stage IV is allowed when stuttering and fluency technique goals are met for three consecutive weeks. Finally, the clients decide the goals appropriate to their needs.

Stage IV: During this stage, the consultations with the clinicians are less frequent. The aim is for clients to self-manage any of the variations of stuttering severity that usually occur during the maintenance phase of treatment. During each interaction with the clinician, the client has to (a) maintain near stutter-free speech throughout the meeting (b) have a confirmed (audio recording) acceptable stuttering severity and fluency technique scores (c) demonstrate ways in which variations of stuttering severity have been dealt with. The client is discharged when the client exhibits the (a) skills to monitor their speech and control their stuttering (b) ability to address variations in the severity of stuttering and is able to (c) achieve personalized goals for the stuttering treatment.

Adaptation of Camperdown Programme to Telerehabilitation Mode

Camperdown programme can be delivered through the following two modalities.

1. Synchronous delivery mode: The concept and the treatment stages of traditional Camperdown programme will remain the same except the treatment delivery mode which is done through webcam with few adaptations: (a) the treatment was delivered through video teleconferencing/telephone [Skype], (b) one on one clinician and patient interaction during treatment, (c) treatment was provided once a week approximately, (d) no clinic attendance, (e) duration of the treatment varied from 30 to 60 minutes depending on the availability of the clinician and the participant and (f) parents involvement varied depending upon the age of the participants.

Technological support required for telerehabilitation is a computer with webcam, Internet connection with good speed, headphones and Skype software.

2. Asynchronous delivery mode: All the prerecorded prolonged speech technique exemplar videos and descriptions, clinical materials (rating scales) and instructions were uploaded to the linked administration website or mailed individually. These materials are made available electronically to the client and the clinician monitored the patient's activity log. An email reminder was sent to the participants to follow the steps of the intervention programme.

All the participants in both the mode were instructed to send a recorded speech sample via e-mail/designated telephone voicemail for stuttering analysis. Few studies adapting Camperdown programme via telemode are given below.

O'Brian, Packman and Onslow (2008) carried out a Phase I trial study to investigate the feasibility of telehealth delivery of the Camperdown programme to treat adults who stutter. Ten participants were recruited for the study, who were unable to attend regular therapy during working hours. All the participants have treated via synchronous delivery mode by the clinician-client contact remotely through email and telephone. All the participants completed the programme and the results revealed a reduction of 82 per cent in stuttering frequency immediately after the treatment. A reduction of the stuttering frequency of about 74 per cent was reported after six months during the follow-up. However, participants exhibited significant individual variations in response to the telehealth delivery of the Camperdown programme. These findings suggest that telehealth Camperdown programme is efficient and has the potential to treat stuttering in individuals who cannot afford traditional face-to-face therapy.

Carey et al. (2010) studied whether the telehealth Camperdown programme can be an alternative to traditional face-to-face intervention for adults who stutter. This study included a parallel-group; non-inferiority randomized controlled trial with multiple blinded outcome assessments. Forty adults whom stutters were recruited for the study were randomized: 20 were randomly allotted to face-to-face arm and telehealth arm (synchronous mode) respectively. In both the intervention modalities Camperdown treatment programme for adults was implemented. The primary outcome measures of stuttering included the percentage of syllable stuttered and the total number of intervention hours. The secondary outcome measures included self-reported stuttering severity, treatment satisfaction and speech naturalness. Results revealed that there was no clinically or statistically significant difference in the percentage of syllables stuttered between the two groups even after nine months post-randomization. Analysis of covariance of the baseline percentage of syllables stuttered reflected a 0.8 per cent fewer syllables stuttered in telehealth mode in comparison to face-to-face arm. However, there was no significant difference in the percentage of syllable stuttered during follow-ups between the groups. Also, the time consumed by telehealth mode was statistically lesser on an average when compared to the face-to-face arm. These shreds of evidence suggest that Camperdown programme can be delivered through telehealth mode as an alternative to traditional face-to-face mode to treat adults who stutter.

Carey et al. (2012) conducted a Phase I trial study to explore the practicability in implementing webcam delivery model using Camperdown programme to treat adolescents who stutter. Three participants with the age range between 13 and 16 years with moderate to severe stuttering were employed for the study. Each of the participants was treated using Camperdown treatment programme via the synchronous delivery mode (webcam-Skype). Results revealed that a mean of 18 sessions and 11 clinician hours were required to reach the maintenance phase. Group mean per cent SS score of the experiment group in post-treatment was 83 per cent and 93 per cent at six months follow up and 74 per cent at 12 months follow-up. Self-reported stuttering severity ratings were in consensus with these results. Telerehabilitation using Camperdown programme was effective in treating adolescents with stuttering. These results warrant a detailed Phase II trial study of the delivery mode.

Carey et al. (2014) conducted a Phase II study to investigate the responsiveness of adolescents who stutter to the webcam delivered Camperdown programme (synchronous delivery mode). To meet the aim of the study, sixteen adolescents were recruited for the study. All the participants were treated using Camperdown programme through webcam without clinic attendance. The primary stuttering outcome measures considered are the percentage of stuttering syllables and secondary outcome measures included the number of hours, weeks and sessions to maintenance, speech satisfaction, self-reported stuttering severity, self-reported anxiety, speech naturalness, the self-reported impact of stuttering, self-reported situation avoidance and satisfaction with webcam treatment delivery. Data was collected pre-treatment and post 12 months of treatment. Fourteen participants completed the treatment programme. The pre-treatment group mean stuttering frequency was 6.11 per cent syllables stuttered and the 12 months post-treatment score was 2.8 per cent syllables stuttered after entering into maintenance. Besides, half of the participants mean score was 1.2 per cent syllables stuttered or even lesser during the maintenance phase. All the participants completed the treatment programme with a mean of 25 sessions (15.5 hours). The obtained results were in consensus with self-reported stuttering impact scores, speech satisfaction scores and self-reported stuttering severity ratings. Minimal anxiety was observed in both pre- and post-treatment. However, participants exhibited individual variations in responses to treatment with half of the participants revealing a little reduction in speech situation avoidance. Participants found the webcam service delivery model to be more desirable. However, it was effective and efficient only for half of the participants.

Erickson et al. (2016) conducted a clinician free Internet-based stuttering treatment delivered through asynchronous mode for adults who stutter. The speech restructuring consisted of nine phases, which was loosely based on Camperdown programme. 20 adults with stuttering were employed for the study for six months with unlimited access to the programme. The primary outcome measures of stuttering include the percentage of syllable stuttered and self-perceived stuttering severity ratings. Only five participants accessed all the phases while another five participants accessed more than half of the phases and remaining 10 participants accessed from one to four phases. Results revealed that the participants who accessed all the phases witnessed a reduction in stuttering frequency by 50 per cent and similar results were observed in two participants who accessed more than half of the treatment phases. These results were in consensus with the self-perceived stuttering severity ratings. These results were significantly proportional to the number of treatment phases accessed by the participants. If the participants maintain the adherence to the treatment programme procedures, the stuttering reduction can be significant, which is the primary concern in all clinician free treatment programmes. However, this new approach to treat stuttering may help some clients as an alternative treatment mode and further detailed research is required to address relapse and access issues in this treatment modality which might lead to poor prognosis.

Integrated Approach

The integrated approach is also known as 'hybrid' Intervention. It is the combination of various features of the different intervention approaches. Few authors titled such blended intervention programme as 'integrative' approach (Guitar 2013). These programmes have been used in traditional therapy, which has shown a considerable gain in both cognitive/affective and fluency measures. Hasbrouck (1992) treated 117 adults who stuttered with the integrative approach, which involves Electromyographic biofeedback, desensitization, progressive relaxation and airflow management. He reported that all the participants met the one per cent stuttered words discharge criteria and 42 of them maintained the fluency.

Intensive treatment programmes predominantly combine the characteristics of cognitive behavioural therapy and fluency shaping. The well-known and better-documented intervention programme, which uses an integrated approach, is the Comprehensive Stuttering Therapy (CST) (Kully, Langevin and Lomheim 2007; Langevin et al. 2006). CST is conducted at the Institute of Stuttering Treatment and Research (ISTAR), Canada.

Adaptation of the Integrated Approach to Telerehabilitation Mode

Teletreatment was delivered by combining different intervention approaches through synchronous mode only, with few modifications such as (a) Inclusion of videoconferencing via Skype to deliver the intervention, (b) employing videoconferencing to carry out follow-up telepractice, after the completion of traditional direct intervention, (c) utilizing email facility to communicate between clinician and participants in addition to the traditional integrated approach to enhance effectiveness of communication, counselling and follow-ups.

For all the participants in tele-practice mode, speech samples were obtained via real-time online videoconferencing for stuttering analysis. Few studies adapted to integrated approach via telemode are given below.

A preliminary study was done by Kully (2000) to investigate the applicability of telemedicine for the treatment of stuttering. A 38-year-old individual with severe developmental stuttering from rural telehealth centre participated in the study through videoconferencing. The participant had completed a three-week intensive treatment and was currently in a follow-up programme. The telehealth rehabilitative sessions were given for two months with each session lasting for an hour by providing practice on specific speech skills, strategies, problem-solving and self-management skills. Feedback was given through visual or verbal modality. Outcome measures were reported based on the informal report from the participant and the clinician, which showed a positive outcome. Thus, the authors postulated that, if this form of rehabilitation is found to be successful and cost-effective in future, it might be used as an effective form of treatment especially for children in early intervention stages.

Allen (2011) studied 16 clients between the age range of 19 to 52 years, with the covert and overt symptoms ranging from mild to severe, who participated in the study. The intervention programme employed was devised mainly on individual presentation of stuttering, blending of different speech modification techniques and counselling via both face-to-face appointments as well as an email exchange. The authors report the email to serve two purposes, one being administrative and the other being therapeutic. Total 328 emails (69%) were exchanged in arranging for appointments and 144 (31%) emails were exchanged in monitoring existing treatment goals and also in offering problem-solving guidance, adding up to 472 emails containing administrative and therapeutic information. The benefits gained through email were reported to being able to improve access to the available services, improving the clinical decision-making, enabling lasting personal growth, supporting the speech change, matching the therapist-client relationship and enhancing caseload management. The authors highlight that even though email can be used for therapy, the effectiveness and ethics, the rationale for the clinical practice involving the telemode -email need careful monitoring. Email can lead to misinterpretation of information when client gives poor attention to the message. For instances, repeated reading of the same email may present a new meaning with each time of reading. In cases where the client is restricted to exclusive email therapy, there is room for misinterpretation of the intended information compared to a face-to-face set-up. There is also the scope of uncertainty in emails as to if the client has overlooked/forgotten to check emails, been too busy to check, is no longer involved in therapy or whether practical/technical difficulties have prevented the client from accessing emails.

Irani and Gabel (2011) reported a case study in which they described the positive outcomes of an intensive intervention programme for a 21-year-old adult who stutters. This eclectic approach was implemented by combining an intensive stuttering programme in traditional face-to-face mode and 12 months follow up through video telepractice. The participants received three weeks (75 hours) of intensive therapy with non-intensive follow-up sessions through video telepractice. The results revealed a positive effect on the participant's fluency skills, which reflected in the reduction of the percentage of syllables stuttered, stuttering severity ratings and a positive change in feelings and attitude towards stuttering and speaking situations. Overall, the follow-ups done via video telepractice enhanced the effectiveness of the intensive traditional therapy for this participant. This method was cost-effective and efficient, considering the amount of real-time and money required for the follow ups the geographical locations.

Valentine (2015) focused on studying three different delivery models, that are, direct, hybrid and telepractice for two 11-year-old children with a moderate degree of stuttering. Intervention programme comprised of stuttering modification protocol and modification of smooth easy speech which was delivered through direct, hybrid and telemode. The authors used the outcome measures as a parameter in understanding different models and also aimed to examine if short-term goals were preserved across the telepractice sessions of the client. The outcome measures considered were: Stuttering Severity Instrument, Fourth Edition (SSI-4) along with which weekly fluency samples (percentage of stuttered syllables in a monologue) were attained over a 10-week intervention period. The Communication Attitudes Test (Revised) was also additionally administered to measure the children's attitude to speaking. Post the telepractice period, parents and children were administered a questionnaire concerning the therapy experience via telepractice. The results obtained via the outcome measures, post the 10-week programme, showed varied outcomes, the severity ratings remained consistent for one client and the other child showed improvement in the rating scores; thus, the authors concluded the study by stating that the telepractice is a viable mode which can be used in improving and maintaining fluency in individuals with fluency disorders.

Eslami Jahromi and Ahmadian (2018) explored the infrastructure required for the implementation of telemedicine and studied the therapeutic satisfaction of persons who stutter concerning the method used. Thirty persons who stutter between 14 and 39 years underwent speech therapy sessions through videoconferencing via Skype. The data collection tool was a researcher-made questionnaire consisting of four sections. Section I comprised the demographic information; questions regarding the satisfaction of the infrastructure available to delivering the telespeech therapy was covered in section II. Section III consisted of questioning pertaining to the patient's satisfaction with respect to the treatment method used, and the final section consisted of three open-ended questions regarding the advantages and disadvantages of a remote treatment method compared to a face-to-face method with the preferred method. The results obtained from the data showed no significant relationship between client's satisfaction and demographic data, that are, the gender, education level and age. The number of speech therapy sessions also did not affect the overall satisfaction of the patients. However, it was reported that the number of therapeutic sessions undergone by the client had a direct impact on the satisfaction with the infrastructure used for telespeech therapy. The authors concluded the study by stating that patients were satisfied with telespeech therapy but the low speed of the Internet connection in the country was a major challenge for receiving telespeech therapy.

SUMMARY

For the present chapter, 15 articles were identified: five articles about Camperdown programme; five articles addressing the Lidcombe programme and another five articles concerning the integrated approach. The studies included different research designs such as Phase I, Phase II clinical trials and randomized control clinical trials. Phase I clinical trials are the preliminary investigations of a new treatment, conducted on only a few participants who may be volunteers. The primary consideration of Phase I trials are safety and viability from the perspective of the client and the service provider. The primary considerations during this stage of the trial are to establish estimates of how many participants will respond to the treatment. Randomized control trials are done when subjects are randomly assigned to one of the two groups. One is the experimental group receiving the intervention that is being presently tested, another being the control group receiving an alternative form of treatment. The two different groups are followed up to see if there is any difference in the outcome measures.

Tele-Lidcombe Programme: Phase I Trials

Summarizing the evidence on telerehabilitation using Lidcombe programme suggests that this programme has proven to yield better parent satisfaction and is beneficial, comfortable, convenient, reliable, efficient and cost-effective for treating children with stuttering who have limited access to standard delivery of the Lidcombe programme. Thus, the webcam treatment to be better than the only telephone-based Lidcombe programme for children who have limited access to the clinically based standard programme. Wilson, Onslow and Lincoln (2004) also suggested that the distant delivery of the Lidcombe programme would be more efficient if further supplemented with videoconferencing.

Camperdown Programme via Videoconferencing

Summarizing the evidence on telerehabilitation using Camperdown programme suggests that it is effective in treating adolescents with stuttering. However, it is essential that the participants maintain the adherence to the treatment programme procedures, due to which there would be a significant reduction in stuttering. Also, the time consumed by telehealth mode is found to be statistically lesser on an average when compared to the face-to-face arm. The evidence that is mentioned above suggests that Camperdown programme can be delivered through telehealth mode to treat adults who stutter as an alternative to traditional face-to-face mode. Carey and his colleagues also suggest the telehealth version of the Camperdown programme to be efficient and to be full of potential to treat stuttering in individuals who cannot afford traditional face-to-face therapy (Carey et al. 2012). Similarly, Phase II clinical trial results also suggest that the webcam service delivery model was desirable by the participants (Carey et al. 2014). However, it was effective and efficient only for half of the participants.

Integrated Approach via Telepractice

On the whole, the researchers conclude that an integrated approach to be recommended for individuals with stuttering. The outcomes observed demonstrate that telepractice is viable for improving and maintaining fluency. Overall, the follow ups done via video telepractice enhanced the effectiveness of the intensive traditional therapy for the participant. This could be due to the reduced cost and avoiding the travel time towards the follow ups.

MERITS AND DEMERITS OF TELEREHABILITATION IN STUTTERING

As technology advances, it helps the professionals immensely to reach the unreached patients; however, there are some issues, which need to be addressed for better effectiveness of the telehealth service delivered.

Merits of Telerehabilitation in Stuttering

1. Trained SLPs can deliver the service for the patients who hail from remote areas where traditional therapy is difficult, primarily rural areas.
2. Trained SLPs can address a larger group of patients, in turn, reducing the waiting period at the clinics.
3. Telepractice is economical in terms of transportation cost and time.
4. Traditional therapy, combined with telepractice for follow up, has proven to maintain better fluency skills.
5. Telehealth service delivery is more convenient for the working class and students who cannot attend the traditional therapy during working hours; thus increasing the number of patients receiving the intervention.

Demerits of Telerehabilitation in Stuttering

1. Telepractice requires an excellent Internet connection and updated computers to deliver the service, which may be a hurdle in developing and underdeveloped countries.
2. It was also observed that the patients were satisfied with telespeech therapy; however, the low speed of the Internet connection in the country was a significant challenge for receiving telespeech therapy.
3. Patients are expected to have the necessary knowledge on how to use computer and Internet facilities, which may pose as a barrier in a specific population.
4. It was also noted that in a few cases, the gain observed was less and the maintenance was also inadequate because patients fail to follow the procedures and instructions of the intervention programme.
5. The success of telepractice is questioned if the risk of privacy and security is not addressed because telepractice involves lack of control over the use of collected data and disclosure of sensitive personal information.

CONCLUSION

A total of 15 articles were presented in this chapter and from the results, it can be concluded that telerehabilitation using Lidcombe programme, Camperdown programme and the integrated programme are effective in treating an individual with stuttering. Several Phase I studies, followed by Phase II studies and randomized control trials were conducted in this regard. In telepractice, it is essential that the participants maintain the adherence to the treatment programme procedures, due to which there would be a significant reduction in stuttering. Studies also report the time consumed by telehealth mode to be statistically lesser compared to the face-to-face arm. Evidence also suggests these programmes can be delivered through telehealth mode to treat individuals who stutter as an alternative to traditional face-to-face mode. Telepractice has also proved to yield better parent satisfaction, as it is beneficial, comfortable, convenient, reliable, efficient, and cost-effective for treating children with stuttering, who may have limited access to standard delivery of the programme.

INDIAN SCENARIO

In the past decade, India has witnessed enormous growth in the field of digitalization. With the advancement of digital resources available in India, there is a need to launch telepractice to provide evidence-based intervention programmes on a larger scale. There are only a few reports available at AIISH telecentre, which are based on case studies of children with the autism spectrum disorder, children with disfluency, Wernicke's aphasia and other conditions (Goswami, Bhutada and Jayachandran 2012). It can be construed from these studies that telepractice through both hybrid (a combination of face-to-face and virtual treatment) and information and communication technology (ICT) mode provide benefits to the individuals receiving the treatment. Stuttering is one of the speech motor disorders that might require rehabilitation for a longer duration. There is a dearth in information and efforts, to meet the requirements of our unique multilingual population except for few documented tests and web resources (e.g., Aphasia Corner, Boardmaker® Online and Constant Therapy).

However, even with the advancement of ICT (such as emails, multimedia content, videoconferencing, Skype, Google group, Team Viewer, and other interactive dedicated software), a few prerequisites need to be fulfilled for launching telepractice on a large scale. The primary considerations would be regarding the availability of validated digital resources for assessment and therapeutic services through telepractice, professional skills and code of ethics regarding telepractice. Another primary concern would be regarding the privacy issues of both, the person providing treatment and the individual receiving the treatment. Further, there is a dearth of literature regarding the different modes of service delivery and their outcome, which needs to be undertaken to establish the efficacy of using telepractice.

REFERENCES

Allen, Carolyn R. 2011. 'The Use of Email as a Component of Adult Stammering Therapy: A Preliminary Report.' *Journal of Telemedicine and Telecare* 17 (4): 163–167. doi: 10.1258/jtt.2010.100114

Bridgman, Kate, Mark Onslow, Susan O'Brian, Mark Jones, and Susan Block. 2016. 'Lidcombe Program Webcam Treatment for Early Stuttering: A Randomized Controlled Trial.' *Journal of Speech, Language, and Hearing Research* 59 (5): 932–939.

Carey, Brenda, Sue O Brian, Mark Onslow, Ann Packman, and Ross Menzies. 2012. 'Webcam Delivery of the Camperdown Program for Adolescents Who Stutter: A Phase I Trial.' *The ASHA Leader* 43 (3): 370–380. Available at: https://doi: 10.1044/0161-1461(2011/11-0010)

Carey, Brenda, Sue O'Brian, Robyn Lowe, and Mark Onslow. 2014. 'Webcam Delivery of the Camperdown Program for Adolescents Who Stutter: A Phase II Trial.' *Language, Speech, and Hearing Services in Schools* 45 (4): 314–324.

Carey, Brenda, Sue O'Brian, Mark Onslow, Susan Block, Mark Jones, and Ann Packman. 2010. 'Randomized Controlled Non-Inferiority Trial of a Telehealth Treatment for Chronic Stuttering: The Camperdown Program.' *International Journal of Language and Communication Disorders* 45 (1): 108–120. doi: 3109/13682820902763944

Cherney, Leora R, and Sarel Van Vuuren. 2012. 'Telerehabilitation, Virtual Therapists, and Acquired Neurologic Speech and Language Disorders.' *Seminars in Speech and Language* 33 (3): 243–258.

Craig, Ashley, Karen Hancock, Yvonne Tran, Magali Craig, and Karen Peters. 2002. 'Epidemiology of Stuttering in the Community across the Entire Life Span.' *Journal of Speech, Language, and Hearing Research* 45 (6): 1097–1105.

Efstathiou, G. 2009. 'Students' Psychological Web Consulting: Function and Outcome Evaluation.' *British Journal of Guidance & Counselling* 37 (3): 243–255.

Erickson, Shane, Susan Block, Ross Menzies, Sue O'Brian, Ann Packman, and Mark Onslow. 2016. 'Standalone Internet Speech Restructuring Treatment for

Adults Who Stutter: A Phase I Study.' *International Journal of Speech-Language Pathology* 18 (4): 329–340. doi: 10.3109/17549507.2015.1101156

Eslami Jahromi, Maryam, and Leila Ahmadian. 2018. 'Evaluating Satisfaction of Patients with Stutter Regarding the Tele-Speech Therapy Method and Infrastructure.' *International Journal of Medical Informatics* 115 (March): 128–133. doi: 10.1016/j.ijmedinf.2018.03.004

Franken, Marie Christine. 1987. 'Perceptual and Acoustic Evaluation of Stuttering Therapy.' In *Speech Motor Dynamics in Stuttering*, 285–294. doi: 10.1007/978-3-7091-6969-8_20

Goswami, S. P., Ankita Bhutada, and Kavitha Jayachandran. 2012. 'Telepractice in a Person with Aphasia.' *Journal of the All India Institute of Speech and Hearing* 31: 159–167.

Guitar, Barry. 2013. *Stuttering: An Integrated Approach to Its Nature and Treatment.* Philadelphia, PA: Lippincott Williams & Wilkins.

Guttormsen, Linn Stokke, Elaina Kefalianos, and Kari Anne B. Næss. 2015. 'Communication Attitudes in Children Who Stutter: A Meta-Analytic Review.' *Journal of Fluency Disorders* 46: 1–14. doi: 10.1016/j.jfludis.2015.08.001

Harrison, Elisabeth, Linda Wilson, and Mark Onslow. 1999. 'Distance Intervention for Early Stuttering with the Lidcombe Programme.' *International Journal of Speech-Language Pathology* 1 (1): 31–36. doi: 10.3109/14417049909167151

Hasbrouck, Jon M. 1992. 'FAMC Intensive Stuttering Treatment Program: Ten Years of Implementation.' *Military Medicine* 157 (5): 244–247.

Hull, F. M., P. W. Mielke, J. A. Willeford, and R. J. Timmons. 1976. *National Speech and Hearing Survey.* Final Report, Project No. 50978, Grant No. OE-32-15-0050-5010 (607). Washington, DC: Office of Education, DHEW.

Irani, Farzan, and Rodney Gabel. 2011. 'Intensive Stuttering Therapy with Telepractice Follow-up: A Case Study.' *Perspectives on Fluency and Fluency Disorders* 21 (1): 11–21.

Iverach, Lisa, Mark Jones, Lauren F. McLellan, Heidi J. Lyneham, Ross G. Menzies, Mark Onslow, and Ronald M. Rapee. 2016. 'Prevalence of Anxiety Disorders among Children Who Stutter.' *Journal of Fluency Disorders* 49: 13–28. doi: 10.1016/j.jfludis.2016.07.002

Johnson, Kia N., Tedra A. Walden, Edward G. Conture, and Jan Karrass. 2010. 'Spontaneous Regulation of Emotions in Preschool Children Who Stutter: Preliminary Findings.' *Journal of Speech, Language, and Hearing Research* 53 (6): 1478–1495.

Jones, Mark, Mark Onslow, Ann Packman, Shelley Williams, Tika Ormond, Ilsa Schwarz, and Val Gebski. 2005. 'Randomised Controlled Trial of the Lidcombe Programme of Early Stuttering Intervention.' *Bmj* 331 (7518): 659.

Koushik, Sarita, Rosalee Shenker, and Mark Onslow. 2009. 'Follow-up of 6–10-Year-Old Stuttering Children after Lidcombe Program Treatment: A Phase I Trial.' 34: 279–290. doi: 10.1016/j.jfludis.2009.11.001

Kully, Deborah. 2000. 'Telehealth in Speech Pathology: Applications to the Treatment of Stuttering.' *Journal of Telemedicine and Telecare* 6 (2_supp.): 39–41. doi: 10.1258/1357633001935509

Kully, Deborah. 2002. 'Venturing into Telehealth: Applying Interactive Technologies to Stuttering Treatment.' *The ASHA Leader* 7 (11): 1–15.

Kully, Deborah, Marilyn Langevin, and Holly Lomheim. 2007. 'Intensive Treatment of Adolescents and Adults Who Stutter.' *Stuttering and Related Disorders of Fluency*, 213–232.

Langevin, Marilyn, Wendy J. Huinck, Deborah Kully, Herman F. M. Peters, Holly Lomheim, and Marian Tellers. 2006. 'A Cross-Cultural, Long-Term Outcome Evaluation of the ISTAR Comprehensive Stuttering Program across Dutch and Canadian Adults Who Stutter.' *Journal of Fluency Disorders* 31 (4): 229–256.

Lewis, Christine, Ann Packman, Mark Onslow, Judy M. Simpson, and Mark Jones. 2008. 'A Phase II Trial of Telehealth Delivery of the Lidcombe Program of Early Stuttering Intervention.' *American Journal of Speech-Language Pathology* 17 (2): 139–149.

O'Brian, Sue, Ann Packman, and Mark Onslow. 2008. 'Telehealth Delivery of the Camperdown Program for Adults Who Stutter: A Phase I Trial.' *Journal of Speech, Language, and Hearing Research* 51 (1): 184–195.

O'Brian, Sue, Brenda Carey, Robyn Lowe, Mark Onslow, Ann Packman, and Angela Cream. 2016. 'The Camperdown Program Stuttering Treatment Guide.' *Australian Stuttering Research Centre*.

O'Brian, Sue, Kylie Smith, and Mark Onslow. 2014. 'Webcam Delivery of the Lidcombe Program for Early Stuttering: A Phase I Clinical Trial.' *Journal of Speech, Language, and Hearing Research* 57 (3): 825–830.

Onslow, Mark, Cheryl Andrews, and Michelle Lincoln. 1994. 'A Control/ Experimental Trial of an Operant Treatment for Early Stuttering.' *Journal of Speech, Language, and Hearing Research* 37 (6): 1244–1259.

Onslow, Mark, Margaret Webber, Elisabeth Harrison, Simone Arnott, Kate Bridgman, Brenda Carey, and W Lloyd. 2017. 'The Lidcombe Program Treatment Guide.' Available at: http://lidcombeprogram.org/wp-content/uploads/2018/03/Lidcombe-Program-Treatment-Guide-December-2017-2.pdf (accessed on 19 December 2019).

Ratner, Nan Bernstein, and Stacy Silverman. 2000. 'Parental Perceptions of Children's Communicative Development at Stuttering Onset.' *Journal of Speech, Language, and Hearing Research* 43 (5): 1252–1263.

Richards, Derek, and Noemi Viganó. 2013. 'Online Counseling: A Narrative and Critical Review of the Literature.' *Journal of Clinical Psychology* 69 (9): 994–1011.

Theodoros, Deborah G. 2008. 'Telerehabilitation for Service Delivery in Speech-Language Pathology.' *Journal of Telemedicine and Telecare* 14 (5): 221–224. doi: 10.1258/jtt.2007.007044

Valentine, Daniel T. 2015. 'Stuttering Intervention in Three Service Delivery Models (Direct, Hybrid, and Telepractice): Two Case Studies.' *International Journal of Telerehabilitation* 6 (2): 51–64. doi: 10.5195/IJT.2014.6154

Wilson, Linda, Mark Onslow, and Michelle Lincoln. 2004. 'Telehealth Adaptation of the Lidcombe Program of Early Stuttering Intervention.' *American Journal of Speech-Language Pathology* 13 (1): 81–92.

Yairi, Ehud, and Nicoline Grinager Ambrose. 2005. *Early Childhood Stuttering.* Austin: Pro-Ed Inc.

Yairi, Ehud, and Carol Hibbord Seery. 2015. *Stuttering: Foundations and Clinical Applications.* Upper Saddle River, NJ: Pearson.

Tele-audiology in India

Facilitators, Limitations and Challenges

Saransh Jain, Chandni Jain, Vijaya Kumar Narne and Hemanth N. Shetty

INTRODUCTION

Telehealth is described as the use of telecommunication technologies to deliver health-related services and information that support patient care, administrative activities and health education (Dixon, Hook and McGowan 2008). Telemedicine is defined as providing medical services over distance (Fong, Li and Fong 2013). There is a growing amount of literature on the use of technology for remote assessment and intervention in medicine (Bashshur 2002) and rehabilitation (Lemaire, Boudrias and Greene 2001; Torsney 2003; Winters 2002). Remote areas often have a shortage of professionals and technical resources, which are required for the delivery of services in the specialized medical fields (Callas, Ricci and Caputo 2000). These shortages in professionals negatively affect both health care providers and patients. Rural health care providers are often isolated from medical advancements and technologies used in more substantial metropolitan centres. As a result, when people in rural areas need assessment and/or specific treatment, they may have to travel long distances to get specialized healthcare required to address their needs. To address these problems of the rural and under-accessed population, technologists and clinicians have explored the use of telecommunication and information technologies as a way of bridging the gap among individuals in remote areas who require specialized medical services and the source of specialty care (Benschoter, Wittson and Ingham 1965; Heinzelmann, Lugn and Kvedar 2005).

American Speech-Language-Hearing Association (ASHA) uses the term 'telepractice' to refer to 'the application of telecommunications technology to deliver professional services at a distance' (American Speech-Language-Hearing Association 2014). Since 1998, ASHA has studied the potential impact of telepractice on speech-language pathologists (SLPs) and audiologists and the individuals they serve. ASHA has published a formal position statement, various technical reports and issue briefs that summarize evidence about the use of telepractice in audiology and discusses future directions and research.

The tele-audiology services have various advantages which include increasing patient access to healthcare services (Hofstetter et al. 2010), cost-effective services, reduced inconvenient travels (Smith et al. 2003) and minimizes the stress of caregivers who provide transportation to appointments (Chiang et al. 2012). Tele-interventions also improve functional independence in older adults with chronic illnesses (Chumbler et al. 2004) and have shown to be successful for the treatment of older adults with mobility impairments (Sanford et al. 2007). Teleservices are offered either in asynchronous (stored and later forwarded to audiologist site), synchronous (real-time), remote monitoring, and remote monitoring–interactive models.

In *asynchronous model,* the disease data of the client is collected and the data is stored at the remote site. This data is later forwarded to the consultant professional for diagnosis and further recommendations. Here the facilitator directs the client's involvement. In *synchronous model,* real-time interaction between the clinician and the client is present, leading to face-to-face service using desktop-sharing software (e.g., TeamViewer). A facilitator follows the professional's instructions. *Remote monitoring* is a model of telepractice, which is usually used for rehabilitation purposes, especially in training. A training module, as part of the standardized therapy programme, is provided either online or as a downloadable version. The clinician monitors the performed activity and gives feedback, if necessary. For effective implementation of the programme, any family member or caregiver can aid the client. In this programme, the involvement of the facilitator is optional. *Remote monitoring interaction* model is carried out in training or programming of client's own medical devices. In this method, the clinician continuously monitors the session, provides the feedback and recommends the future goals or the steps to be taken. Based on the feedback given by the clinician, the family members/ caregiver can change the therapy provided to the client. In this programme, the involvement of facilitator is optional. The most effective and efficient service delivery is the **hybrid model**, where the service is delivered by the use of both asynchronous and synchronous models (Swanepoel 2013).

TELE-ASSESSMENT IN AUDIOLOGY

Telepractice in audiology can be used for diagnostic audiology, remote hearing aid fittings and real-time rehabilitation. Audiologists use the opportunity of telecommunication systems to offer remote hearing services to individuals around the world where physical access to the professionals is challenging. Audiologists and patients must also willingly accept tele-audiology for it to become mainstream. Studies in tele-audiology have focused on its use for answering patients' questions and for counselling. Singh (2014) reported that the patients' point of views were positive on tele-audiology, with about 75 per cent of patients being moderate to extremely willing to try tele-audiology. Cohn and Cason (2012) had also reported that many audiological services might be delivered through telepractice.

Yao et al. (2015) had developed a browser-server-based tele-audiology system for pure tone audiometry and speech audiometry. The system has a web application server, an embedded Internet-Bluetooth gateway, and a Bluetooth-enabled audiometer. Several graphical user interfaces and a relational database were also hosted on the application server. The system was in a console device that was designed to run the tests and communication between the local site and the remote site. The data was collected at an audiology laboratory and the results showed that pure-tone audiogram and speech test results were comparable with the results obtained from the conventional face-to-face approach. Angley, Schnittker and Tharpe (2017) had evaluated the benefits of remote audiological follow-up care. The researchers had reported that 82 per cent of patients were able to install software with no assistance and 60 per cent preferred remote appointments in future over face-to-face appointments.

Smits et al. (2004) have developed a computerized test that can be administered through telephones, which is a test of hearing screening, measuring the speech reception thresholds in the presence of noise. The test is automated and uses digit triplets as the stimuli. They report that the telephone type and listening environment did not have any influence on the thresholds. The authors claim that the sensitivity and the specificity of the test is 0.91 and 0.93, respectively.

Tele-audiology also has the potential for neonatal screening and rehabilitation. It would ensure that infants who require audiology services can receive them in a timely and coordinated manner. Early Hearing Detection and Intervention (EHDI) states that infants should be screened within one month post birth, diagnosed within three months and rehabilitation should be initiated within six months, which is known as the 1–3–6 rule. Unfortunately, many infants who fail in their newborn hearing screening, do not follow up due to the difficulty in accessing an audiologist, which poses a more significant challenge for families living in rural and remote areas. Thus, tele-audiology would be a practical option to conduct diagnostic evaluations with infants who fail in initial hearing screening and may not follow up. Some aspects of audiology, such as behavioural assessments of infants, often require the professional to be in close physical proximity to the client and are not viable through telemode. The use of synchronous impedance testing via telepractice is expected to become more prevalent as computer-based tympanometry continues to be developed (Krumm and Vento 2013).

Mobile phones provide an excellent medium for tele-audiological services and access to mobile phones is rapidly increasing. According to a report from the World Bank, 75 per cent of the world's population uses mobile phones. It was also noted that in Africa, where there is little to no provision of hearing healthcare, there are about 700 million mobile phone users among the one billion who live there. With the advent of technology, these mobile phones can be connected to the Internet. Thus, it is possible for the patient to connect with professionals using various real-time videoconferencing services. These services are available on mobile phones as well as computers, thus making tele-audiology possible through videos. The high-resolution cameras available on smartphones and tablets make it further easy to use, store and forward the videos. Several hearing-related smartphone applications already exist (Bright and Pallawela 2016; Kam et al. 2013; Smits, Kapteyn and Houtgast 2004), which can be downloaded directly through the Internet. Similarly, there are various apps available to test and screen hearing sensitivity for tinnitus assessment (Sereda et al. 2019). However, the users of downloadable hearing screening apps need mechanisms to evaluate the validity of the results they provide and the availability of telephones in the rural set-up is uncommon in India and hence, restricts the usage of this method.

TELEREHABILITATION IN AUDIOLOGY

Clinicians are also accepting remote hearing aid adjustment assessments of new hearing aid users (Singh et al. 2014). Few studies have also assessed the use of telepractice for cochlear implant (CI) service delivery (Franck, Pengelly and Zerfoss 2006; Goehring et al. 2012; Hughes et al. 2012; McElveen et al. 2010; Ramos et al. 2009; Shapiro et al. 2008; Wesarg et al. 2010). Franck and colleagues (2006) were one of the first group of researchers to describe their experiences with CI programming via remote technology, at the Children's Hospital of Philadelphia and described it as a successful process for experienced CI users at their clinic. Similarly, Shapiro and colleagues (2008) used tele-audiology for intraoperative electro-physiological testing during CI surgery. The study focused on the time-saving aspect, which showed that remote testing was considerably more time-efficient for clinicians.

Ramos and colleagues (2009) performed remote programming for five adult recipients of Advanced Bionics (AB) HiRes 90K CIs using a split-half design. Subjects had 4–15 weeks of experience with the CI and took part in both remote and standard (face-to-face) programming sessions. Subjects were randomly assigned either to the remote or standard programme during a 3-month interval. The programming and evaluation process was repeated two-three times over 6–9 months. It was noted that there was no significant difference across subjects for MAP M-levels, sound field thresholds or speech perception between MAPs created in the remote and standard conditions.

Wesarg and colleagues (2010) compared map T-and C-levels for remote versus face-to-face fittings and results showed no significant differences in T-or C-levels between the two fitting methods. Further, subjects and programming audiologists also completed a questionnaire after the conclusion of the study. Results showed that overall subjects and audiologists' feedback were positive; 85.5 per cent of subjects were satisfied with the new remote programme compared to 93 per cent with the local fitting. Audiologists rated the remote session as equally comparable to face-to-face programming for 64 per cent of the sessions.

Tele-audiology, using a smartphone, can be a promising tool in the future, which can be used for hearing aid programming and fine-tuning of hearing aids. Such a system could link audiologists with patients located across the world via secure websites that store audiometric and hearing aid fitting data. Jacobs and Saunders (2014) have reported that the combination of smartphone technology and sophisticated networking apps could enable audiology to perform in a minimally equipped remote clinic by training technicians performing standard diagnostic and hearing fitting procedures using interactive videoconferencing software.

TELE-AUDIOLOGY IN INDIA

Telepractice in audiology is well established in a few upper-middle income and high-income countries, including Brazil, South Africa, United States and Australia. Tele-audiology in India is still not a common practice. India is the second-most populous country in the world, with over 1.21 billion people and has a considerable number of people with communication disabilities (Census of India 2013), out of which five million are hearing impaired. The World Health Organization (WHO) describes the hearing loss as an epidemic and, stated that hearing loss-related disabilities can affect up to 16 per cent of the population. There are 360 million persons in the world (5.3% of the world's population) with hearing loss disabilities (World Health Organization 2011).

The National Sample Survey Organization (Census of India 2013) has reported that in India, there are 291 persons per 1,00,000 of the population with a hearing disability and in rural areas, that is, around 310 persons per 1,00,000 with hearing disabilities. WHO (2011) had reported that in India, there are 10,65,462 inhabitants per audiologist compared to 19,603 inhabitants per audiologist in USA. The figures reflect the acute dearth of trained workforce available in India for the early detection of hearing loss and intervention. However, there is an increase in speech and hearing professionals with 51 training institutions generating human resources in the field of speech and hearing, however, the majority of the trained workforce either opt for higher studies in India or abroad or prefer to work in foreign nations due to better emoluments. Thus, persons with communication disorders do not have access to the professionals due to lack of sufficient number of professionals, the distance that they have to travel and the number of days that they need to spend on rehabilitation. In India, the significant population lives in rural areas, and thus, the existing number of professionals in the field is not enough to cater to the demand.

It was also observed that the majority of speech and hearing professionals are located in major cities, and thus, it is difficult to reach the population in rural areas. Therefore, the rural population is deprived of access to the objective and participative methods of hearing screening due to lack of human resources and non-availability of infrastructure. Long-distance communication medium based assessment and rehabilitation can be considered as a suitable alternative to address the shortage of such workforce. A few examples of these include the use of Information and Communication Technology (ICT) tools such as videoconferencing systems, websites and telephones.

In India, tele-audiology may be used for the job, graduate studies, and continuing education through seminars/conferences. In a review, it has been revealed that about 90 per cent of the audiologists who already practiced tele-audiology were interested in increasing their knowledge and in receiving additional training, while 75 per cent of the audiologists who did not practice tele-audiology were interested in additional training to increase their knowledge. This could be because audiologists who already use tele-audiology are familiar with its advantages and benefits. They might also be in a better position to compare their experience with tele-audiology to face-to-face interaction with the patients. Across the respondents, the preferred means to get additional training were conferences, scientific literature, online courses and websites. Additional training sessions exclusively dealing with tele-audiology might be of benefit to the audiologists to keep themselves updated with the current trends and practices (Ravi et al. 2018).

Tele-assessment and telerehabilitation for persons with speech and language disorders are being tried in India in the recent past; however, related to hearing difficulties, it requires further research. Ali Yavar Jung Institute of Speech and Hearing Disabilities, Mumbai, had started a tele self-assessment programme on the web titled 'Know your hearing through the web' in the year, 2000. The advantage of this programme is that it is validated and the person himself can assess his hearing difficulty. However, this programme evaluates hearing through qualitative assessment using a questionnaire.

Telepractice for clinical service delivery has also been started at the Department of Speech Language and Hearing Sciences at Sri Ramachandra University, Chennai, in 2011. Tele-ABRs were used for diagnostic confirmation of hearing loss after two levels of screening by community workers in 34 villages of Kanchipuram district in Tamil Nadu. ABRs have been obtained using satellite-based mobile-telemedicine-van located approximately one kilometre from hospital campus in the rural site using IP-based systems and compared with face-to-face ABRs. Results showed that there was no significant difference between peak V latency in the two modes (Ramkumar et al. 2013).

An online system for hearing screening was developed by Ajish and Jain (2014) at All India Institute of Speech and Hearing (AIISH) for hearing screening at four pure tone frequencies (500 Hz, 1,000Hz, 2,000 Hz & 4,000 Hz) and four intensity levels (25, 30, 35 and 40 dBHL). In the system, a calibrated stimulus delivery system was interfaced with the output of the laptop containing screening software. The system was validated and the hearing screening was done on 270 ears in different villages around Mysuru district of Karnataka state. Results showed that overall sensitivity and specificity were more than 90 per cent for all the frequencies as compared with the portable audiometer.

The feasibility of telehearing screening in schools was evaluated in one of the towns in South India (Monica et al. 2017). Video otoscopy, pure-tone audiometry (PTA) and distortion product otoacoustic emission (DPOAE) were performed both in-person and in telemode. Telehearing screening was done using either mobile hotspot or dongle connectivity. The in-person and televideo otoscopy correlation was around 87.5–96.4 per cent; between in-person and tele-PTA was 80.64 per cent and between in-person and tele-DPOAE was 83.87 per cent. The study concluded that hearing screening in schools could be performed via telemethod with the help of a schoolteacher as a trained facilitator. Thus, successful implementation of tele-audiological assessment procedures demonstrated by the studies implies that tele-audiology for hearing screening of infants, school-going children and adults in the Indian context has excellent potential. However, these studies were mainly conducted in South India and therefore, replication of the study in other parts of the country is necessary. The rehabilitation process involves not only identifying but also providing suitable intervention, be in terms of providing hearing aids or in terms of listening and speech-language therapy or both. Hence, research in the use of telemodel in the audiologic intervention needs to be explored in the Indian context.

However, for the successful implementation of tele-audiology, Internet connectivity and the availability of personnel at the remote site are essential aspects. Most tele-audiology studies have used the Internet for the implementation of the programme. However, Internet access in the rural areas of India is very restricted and thus, alternate means like IP over satellite needs to be explored.

BARRIERS TO TELE-AUDIOLOGY

Despite the potential benefits associated with the use of telemedicine, it has been reported that more than 75 per cent of telemedicine initiatives failed during the early stage (Berg 1999). Broens et al. (2007) and Hailey and Crowe (2003) had conducted meta-analytic reviews of 45 and 89 telemedicine interventions, to understand the high failure rate and to find out the predictors of successful telemedicine interventions. It was reported that the usability of equipment and associated technologies were essential but not sufficient for the successful execution of telemedicine. The success of any teleservice would also depend on the attitude, perceived usefulness and acceptance of the technology by healthcare professionals and stakeholders (Al-Qirim 2007; Charness, Demiris and Krupinski 2012; Hu et al. 1999; Whitten and Love 2005; Whitten and Mackert 2005; Wootton and Hebert 2001). The persons who were less tech-savvy, particularly in cases where they have to drive much on the technology, were poor candidates for tele-audiology. It is also still a question of whether tele-audiology would be a success in children.

Audiology services are both exciting and demanding. Professionals might feel uncertain about how to practice this new approach during their day-to-day services. Patients may also be hesitant about how to access services remotely. Apprehension to use the technology and apprehension of disrupting personal connections are the barriers that both the clinicians and the patients face. Thus, tele-audiology services will not be suitable for all patients and it is challenging to replace live interactions.

Tele-audiology has barriers that need to be answered before it becomes popular among audiologists. These barriers include lack of facilities/infrastructure, software related issues, the speed of Internet, training in tele-audiology, problems related to reimbursement, the reliability of results, licensure related issues and reduced quality when compared to face-to-face interactions (Molini-Avejonas et al. 2015). These barriers are more in low-income countries compared to high-income countries. In high-income countries, tele-audiology is a success, but in low-income countries, these barriers need to be taken care in order to become a routine clinical practice.

CHALLENGES, SOLUTIONS AND RECOMMENDATIONS IN TELE-AUDIOLOGY

Connectivity and Internet capability show that synchronous or asynchronous model is the most suitable to enable service. Although tele-audiology has been adopted for many years, widespread utilization of this approach is often poor. The service delivery and outcome from the distance mode should be equivalent to the same service provided by the conventional face-to-face model. There are various factors that impede the successful implementation of tele-audiology practice like improper planning, infrastructure costs, handling equipment, reliable outcomes, poor transmission, quality of pictures and sounds, upgradation of equipment with the advancement of technology, environment and calibration factors, inadequate training of facilitators and concerns about privacy. The recommendations for the implementation of successful tele-audiology programme are discussed below:

Planning: Technical factors, organizational factors and business factors are the risk factors in planning, as suggested by Cuyler and Holland (Cuyler and Holland 2012). Technical aspect concerns with reliability of outcomes from an equipment.

In organizational factors, the following questions impact proper planning. Who should be the facilitator? What should be their educational background? How should the facilitators be trained? If training is required, then, what are the skills they are to be trained for and for how long, to ensure effective engagement and commitment? In business, the cost-effectiveness and sustainability of tele-audiology practice are concerned factors. Necessary resources and a realistic budget are the most essential components during the development phase of tele-audiology practice. If the demand for tele-audiology is high with good facilitator commitment, then it results in customer satisfaction. The feedback from the client towards the service and eventually taking the corrective and preventive actions certainly improve quality assurance in delivering services to the needy.

Equipment: The professional body of audiology has come up with guidelines for tele-audiology and specifications for instrumentation to deliver the service. Audiology Australia in 2013 (Audiology Australia 2013) had recommended that guidelines for standard telepractice in audiology should be similar to that of conventional face-to-face methods. The following factors are essential to have telepractice in audiology, similar to that of conventional methods. They are, (a) use of equipment according to the Internet bandwidth (if the Internet speed is low then technology in equipment restricts to only to present the tone but unable to have video conferencing)

(b) constant speed and there should no drop in the network bandwidth so that interruption is minimized and the equipment should be user-friendly on both the facilitator's site (remote) and the testing site.

Information technology personnel: Information technology (IT) professionals support in framework, development and implementation stages to enhance the outcomes and increase confidence in the clinicians to deliver the service. They suggest the organizer regarding the budget concerning infrastructure, especially instruments and setting up of a model of telepractice in audiology service. In addition, the IT professional assists the organizers about the best equipment and recommend the procurement from the company (if proprietary item) or from any local dealer. After installing the equipment, the IT professional gives induction programme to the audiologist and the facilitator on how to use the instrument and how to do basic troubleshooting. With the advancement in time, the adoption of technology is an essential component for quality assurance, thus, IT professional in the team aids in developing the technical knowledge in the clinicians who influence the effectiveness of hearing care.

Testing site: Testing sites to deliver service include a variety of set-ups such as schools, hospitals, primary health care centres, district rehabilitative centres, nursing homes and community health centres. The testing environment should be noise-free for hearing assessment and management. The site should have the best connectivity without any drop in speed during the testing period. The environment site should comply with regulations and policy on space, lighting, furniture, room acoustics, permissible noise level and network connectivity. The listed components on standards in policy vary with the kind of service delivered to the client (screening/diagnostic hearing assessment, hearing aid fitting, programming cochlear implant and listening therapy). It is essential to ensure confidentiality, comfort, safety and privacy during tele-audiology session (American Speech-Language-Hearing Association 2014).

Audiologist/Facilitator/Client: An audiologist should perform a pilot study before the actual programme. The clinician has to collect data on the client's hearing evaluation from conventional face-to-face method and also through the Internet at the site of implementation. The data should be compared to look out for the reliability of the hearing threshold across the frequencies. If the valid thresholds are obtained, the service should be extended at the remote site to endorse the validity of the threshold. Also, the clinician should inform the client on privacy provisions (American Speech-Language-Hearing Association 2014) and orient personal involvement in the remote and the testing sites.

Further, clinicians should come out with the course work/ instructions manual for assessment and rehabilitation. It should explicitly mention the skills to be transferred to the facilitator and the method for the same. It induces confidence in them to participate in the programme. One of the critical factors, for success in telepractice in audiology, is the motivation and commitment of the facilitator at the remote site (Victoor et al. 2012). The selection of facilitators depends on the kind of service they assist in the programme. The factors influencing the effectiveness of the facilitator are: educational background, collegial language, skills to use the equipment, ability to build rapport with the client, basic technical knowledge to troubleshoot simple problems at the remote site and communication skills to convey information to both the client and the clinician. In the client's perceptive, the degree of satisfaction from the service for their problem through telepractice results in aid to the sustainability of the programme.

The factors mentioned above should be carefully considered at the time of implementation of telepractice in audiology to provide access to hearing impaired who are underserved. The evidence of solutions on technological issues, mode of service delivery, training requirements to the facilitators and record-keeping promote the urgency of delivery of hearing care services in remote areas of India.

FUTURE RESEARCH DIRECTIONS

The telepractice in the audiology is required to deliver the service to the underserved population. Individuals with hearing loss from the rural population are unaware of hearing care professionals due to lack of awareness and information. Although a few individuals are aware of the professionals to be consulted, they fail to do so as the hearing professionals are located in metropolitan cities. Beneficiaries in underserved communities often report of difficulty in reaching hearing care professionals because of: (a) loss of wages, (b) waiting time, (c) travel and stay expenses during hearing evaluation and treatment and (d) another person accompanying them as a dependent to convey their intentions (especially older adults). The factors mentioned above induce a lack of motivation and ignorance of hearing loss. If hearing loss is not identified early and treated to the earliest, children show a delay in speech, language and cognition, which reflects in poor academic performance. In case of adults having hearing loss, they have severe problems in social communication and restricted vocational opportunities, which significantly increases unemployment in this cohort. Advancements in technology and global revolution in Internet connectivity and cellular networks make it possible to provide hearing health services through telepractice to reach underserved communities. Remote service is found to be useful as it (a) reduces barriers to access and specialized expertise, (b) is cost-effective and (c) enhance provider productivity and consumer convenience.

PROSPECTIVE PLAN IN TELE-AUDIOMETRY

Software: The computer at the remote audiologist's site is configured with the software designed similar to the control panel of conventional audiometry (Figure 5.1), with the option to control the stimulus and transducer through which thresholds are tracked. The videoconferencing option is also provided so that the remote audiologist can see the client's response and instruct on test procedures, if required. If the Internet connection has high speed, then the videoconferencing option is activated to document client response else client response pad is going to send the signal to the remote audiologist site to decide on the successive presentation of the stimulus.

Hardware: A PC-based audiometer is used to deliver the stimulus to the patient. The audiometer is connected to a computer at the

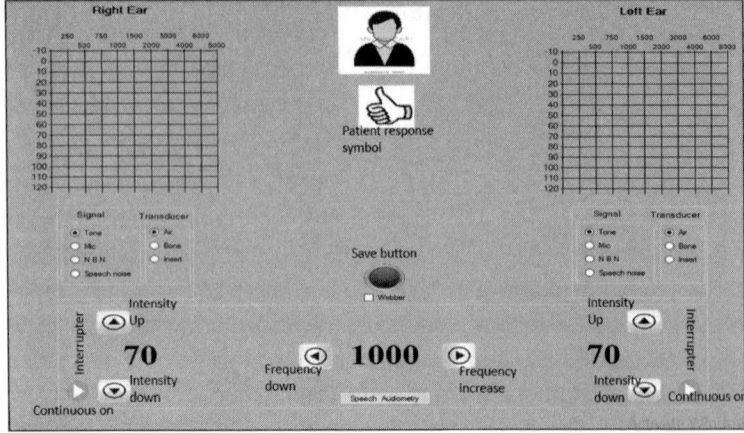

Figure 5.1 *Remote Audiologist Operates the Software Loaded in a Personal Computer*

Source: Screenshot of the unpublished software developed using Visual Studio, at All India Institute of Speech and Hearing, by Hemanth Shetty and Prashanth.

remote site, through internet. The audiometer is comprised of the ethernet port and signal interpreter, and is connected to the internet. The software pre-loaded in computer at remote site sends the information to the audiometer (Figure 5.2). The information is sent through the internet (wired or wireless) to generate the stimuli (a tone/noise of specified frequency and intensity). The audiometer delivers the stimuli to either right or left ear of the patient. The audiometer is equipped to deliver the stimuli either through the air conduction or the bone conduction. The patient response will be sent to the signal interpreter then back to the software (remote site) to decide on the successive presentation of the stimulus. A server connected to the software stores the patient's response for retrieval of data.

Sound booth headphone: A customized headphone is prepared using a noise canceller circuit. The high-fidelity microphone picks up the noise from the site where testing is conducted. The output of the microphone is sent to the digital signal processor. The feedforward active noise cancelling (ANC) algorithm in the digital signal processor and the hardware-oriented Least Mean Square (LMS) algorithm is implemented for the high-performance of ANC

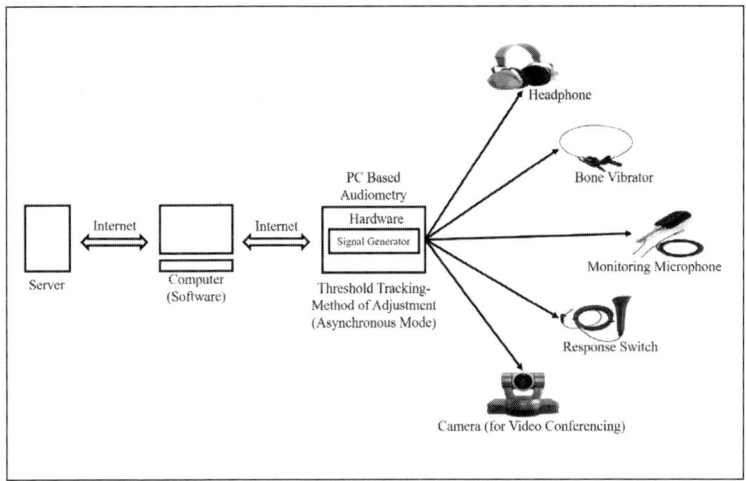

Figure 5.2 *Software Loaded in a Personal System Connects the PC-Based Audiometry through Internet Protocol Connection*

Source: Block diagram of the unpublished software developed using Visual Studio, at All India Institute of Speech and Hearing, by Hemanth Shetty and Prashanth.

algorithm (Chiang et al. 2012). These algorithms cancel the noise if any, in real-time (synchronously). If the noise level is too high, then it will communicate with the software at the remote site to stop the test.

Calibration: The accuracy of generated pure tone for frequency and intensity should be checked for total harmonic distortions (THD), frequency accuracy, rise and fall time and attenuator linearity. The stimulus generated of each frequency is played through the PC-based audiometer. The output is recorded through the B and K sound level meter. The recorded file is transferred to another computer loaded with BZ 5503 software. The transferred files are analysed for THD using either Adobe Audition (version 2) or Matlab file. The pure tone generated from the software is routed to the frequency counter, spectrum analyser, oscilloscope instruments to assess frequency accuracy of pure tone, spectrum (an output level will be displayed as a function of frequency either in a linear or logarithmic scale) and *rise-time and fall-time of waveform (output of the waveform will be displayed as a function of time)*, respectively. Furthermore, the attenuator linearity shall be measured using a multimetre.

Previous literature demonstrated a reliable and valid hearing threshold through telepractice. The development of indigenous products reduce the cost, enabling the organizer to implement telepractice in audiology at a location of the underserved population—the utilization of the developed software aid in performing diagnostic hearing assessment and provide treatment to the beneficiaries.

CONCLUSION

1. Audiology in telepractice, especially for those underserved populations, has an advantage, which eliminates wage loss, waiting period, transportation and other associated costs.
2. Non-audiology facilitators such as village health workers are trained to reduce the burden on audiologists as the hearing care providers are unequally distributed across geography, that is, more in urban areas, less or none in the countryside. Through telehealth, an audiologist can provide services and assess hearing ability of the affected and rehabilitate them through synchronous or asynchronous mode.
3. Installation of frugal innovation of indigenous software and hardware of telehealth in primary health care centres (PHCs: a decentralized clinic) helps to assess hearing ability and to provide treatment in a way such that audiology practice reaches the unreached.
4. Telepractice in audiology (a) reduces the barriers to access services and specialized expertise, (b) is cost-effective and (c) enhance provider's productivity and consumer convenience (e.g., reduce the burden associated with travel time or the costs.

REFERENCES

Ajish, Abraham, and Chandni Jain. 2014. *Development of Online System for Hearing Screening*. All India Institute of Speech and Hearing Research fund DP–114. Mysuru: All India Institute of Speech and Hearing.

Al-Qirim, Nabeel. 2007. 'Championing Telemedicine Adoption and Utilization in Healthcare Organizations in New Zealand.' *International Journal of Medical Informatics* 76 (1): 42–54. doi: 10.1016/j.ijmedinf.2006.02.001

American Speech-Language-Hearing Association. 2014, March. 'Information about Telepractice in Audiology.' Available at: http://www.asha.org/practice/telepractice/.

Angley, Gina P., Jean Anne Schnittker, and Anne Marie Tharpe. 2017. 'Remote Hearing Aid Support: The next Frontier.' *Journal of the American Academy of Audiology* 28 (10): 893–900. doi: 10.3766/jaaa.16093

Audiology Australia. 2013. 'Audiology Australia Professional Practice Standards—Part A Clinical Operations.' Available at: https://audiology.asn.au/Tenant/C0000013/Position%20Papers/Member%20Resources/Part%20A%20Professional%20Practice%20Standards%20-%20Practice%20Operations%20July2013%20EntireDoc.pdf (accessed on 23 December 2019).

Bashshur, R. L. 2002. 'Telemedicine and Health Care.' *Telemedicine Journal and E-Health* 8 (1): 5–12.

Benschoter, Reba Ann, C. L. Wittson, and C. G. Ingham 1965. 'Teaching and Consultation by Television: I. Closed-Circuit Collaboration.' *Mental Hospitals* 16 (3): 99–100.

Berg, M. 1999. 'Patient Care Information Systems and Health Care Work: A Sociotechnical Approach.' *International Journal of Medical Informatics* 55 (2): 87–101.

Bright, Tess, and Danuk Pallawela. 2016. 'Validated Smartphone-Based Apps for Ear and Hearing Assessments: A Review.' *JMIR Rehabilitation and Assistive Technologies* 3 (2): e13. doi:10.2196/rehab.6074

Broens, Tom H. F., Rianne M. H. A. Huis in't Veld, Miriam M. R. Vollenbroek-Hutten, Hermie J. Hermens, Aart T. van Halteren, and Lambert J. M. Nieuwenhuis. 2007. 'Determinants of Successful Telemedicine Implementations: A Literature Study.' *Journal of Telemedicine and Telecare* 13 (6): 303–309. doi: 10.1258/135763307781644951

Callas, P. W., M. A. Ricci, and M. P. Caputo. 2000. 'Improved Rural Provider Access to Continuing Medical Education through Interactive Videoconferencing.' *Telemedicine Journal and E-Health* 6 (4): 393–399. doi: 10.1089/15305620050503861

Census of India. 2013. 'Data On Disability.' Office of the Registrar General & Census Commissioner of India (December). Available at: http://www.disabilityaffairs.gov.in/upload/uploadfiles/files/disabilityinindia2011data.pdf (accessed on 23 December 2019).

Charness, Neil, George Demiris, and Elizabeth A. Krupinski. 2012. *Designing Telehealth for an Aging Population: A Human Factors Perspective.* Human Factors & Aging Series. Boca Raton, FL: Taylor & Francis.

Chiang, Li-Chi, Wan-Chou Chen, Yu-Tzu Dai, and Yi-Lwun Ho. 2012. 'The Effectiveness of Telehealth Care on Caregiver Burden, Mastery of Stress, and Family Function among Family Caregivers of Heart Failure Patients: A Quasi-Experimental Study.' *International Journal of Nursing Studies* 49 (10): 1230–1242. doi: 10.1016/j.ijnurstu.2012.04.013

Chumbler, Neale R., William C. Mann, Samuel Wu, Arlene Schmid, and Rita Kobb. 2004. 'The Association of Home-Telehealth Use and Care Coordination with Improvement of Functional and Cognitive Functioning in Frail Elderly Men.' *Telemedicine Journal and E-Health* 10 (2): 129–137. doi:10.1089/tmj.2004.10.129

Cohn, Ellen R., and Jana Cason. 2012. 'Telepractice: A Wide-Angle View for Persons with Hearing Loss.' *The Volta Review* 112 (3): 207–226. doi: 10.17955/tvr.112.3.m.706

Cuyler, R., and D. Holland. 2012. *Implementing Telemedicine*. Bloomington, IN: Xlibris.

Dixon, B.E, J.M Hook, and J.J McGowan. 2008. 'Using Telehealth to Improve Quality and Safety: Finding from the AHRQ Portfolio.' In *AHRQ Publication No. 09-0012-EF*, 1st ed. Rockville, MD: Agency for Healthcare Research and Quality.

Fong, Bernard, A. C. M. Fong, and C. K. Li. 2013. *Telemedicine Technologies: Information Technologies in Medicine and Telehealth*. Hoboken, NJ: Wiley. Available at: http://rbdigital.oneclickdigital.com (accessed on 1st October 2019)

Franck, K., M. Pengelly, and S. Zerfoss. 2006. 'Telemedicine Offers Remote Cochlear Implant Programming.' *Volta Voices* 13 (1): 16–19.

Goehring, Jenny L., Michelle L. Hughes, Jacquelyn L. Baudhuin, Daniel L. Valente, Ryan W. McCreery, Gina R. Diaz, Todd Sanford, and Roger Harpster. 2012. 'The Effect of Technology and Testing Environment on Speech Perception Using Telehealth with Cochlear Implant Recipients.' *Journal of Speech, Language, and Hearing Research* 55 (5): 1373–1386. doi: 10.1044/1092-4388(2012/11-0358)

Hailey, David, and Bernard Crowe. 2003. 'A Profile of Success and Failure in Telehealth—Evidence and Opinion from the Success and Failures in Telehealth Conferences.' *Journal of Telemedicine and Telecare* 9 (Supp. 2): S22–24.

Heinzelmann, Paul J., Nancy E. Lugn, and Joseph C. Kvedar. 2005. 'Telemedicine in the Future.' *Journal of Telemedicine and Telecare* 11 (8): 384–390. doi: 10.1177/1357633X0501100802

Hofstetter, Philip J., John Kokesh, A. Stewart Ferguson, and Linda J. Hood. 2010. 'The Impact of Telehealth on Wait Time for ENT Specialty Care.' *Telemedicine Journal and E-Health* 16 (5): 551–556. doi: 10.1089/tmj.2009.0142

Hu, Paul J., Patrick Y. K. Chau, Olivia R. Liu Sheng, and Kar Yan Tam. 1999. 'Examining the Technology Acceptance Model Using Physician Acceptance of Telemedicine Technology.' *Journal of Management Information Systems* 16 (2): 91–112. doi: 10.1080/07421222.1999.11518247

Hughes, Michelle L., Jenny L. Goehring, Jacquelyn L. Baudhuin, Gina R. Diaz, Todd Sanford, Roger Harpster, and Daniel L. Valente. 2012. 'Use of Telehealth for Research and Clinical Measures in Cochlear Implant Recipients:

A Validation Study.' *Journal of Speech, Language, and Hearing Research* 55 (4): 1112–1127. doi:10.1044/1092-4388(2011/11-0237)

Jacobs, Peter G., and Gabrielle H. Saunders. 2014. 'New Opportunities and Challenges for Teleaudiology within Department of Veterans Affairs.' *Journal of Rehabilitation Research and Development* 51 (5): vii–xii. doi: 10.1682/JRRD.2014.04.0093

Kam, Anna Chi Shan, Han Gao, Lawrence Kwok Chang Li, Hailian Zhao, ShuqiQiu, and Michael Chi Fai Tong. 2013. 'Automated Hearing Screening for Children: A Pilot Study in China.' *International Journal of Audiology* 52 (12): 855–860. doi: 10.3109/14992027.2013.832419

Krumm, Mark, and Barbara A. Vento. 2013. 'Applications in Teleaudiology.' In *Telerehabilitation*, edited by Sajeesh Kumar and Ellen R. Cohn, 125–138. Health Informatics. London: Springer. doi: 10.1007/978-1-4471-4198-3_9

Lemaire, E. D., Y. Boudrias, and G. Greene. 2001. 'Low-Bandwidth, Internet-Based Videoconferencing for Physical Rehabilitation Consultations.' *Journal of Telemedicine and Telecare* 7 (2): 82–89. doi: 10.1258/1357633011936200.

McElveen, John T., Erin L. Blackburn, J. Douglas Green, Patrick W. McLear, Donald J. Thimsen, and Blake S. Wilson. 2010. 'Remote Programming of Cochlear Implants: A Telecommunications Model.' *Otology & Neurotology* 31 (7): 1035–1040. doi: 10.1097/MAO.0b013e3181d35d87

Molini-Avejonas, Daniela Regina, SilmaraRondon-Melo, Cibelle Albuquerque de La Higuera Amato, and Alessandra Giannella Samelli. 2015. 'A Systematic Review of the Use of Telehealth in Speech, Language and Hearing Sciences.' *Journal of Telemedicine and Telecare* 21 (7): 367–376. doi: 10.1177/1357633X15583215

Monica, Saleth D., Vidya Ramkumar, Mark Krumm, Nitya Raman, Roopa Nagarajan, and Lakshmi Venkatesh. 2017. 'School Entry Level Tele-Hearing Screening in a Town in South India—Lessons Learnt.' *International Journal of Pediatric Otorhinolaryngology* 92 (January): 130–135. doi: 10.1016/j.ijporl.2016.11.021

Ramkumar, Vidya, James W. Hall, Roopa Nagarajan, Vanaja C. Shankarnarayan, and Selvakumar Kumaravelu. 2013. 'Tele-ABR Using a Satellite Connection in a Mobile van for Newborn Hearing Testing.' *Journal of Telemedicine and Telecare* 19 (5): 233–237. doi: 10.1177/1357633X13494691

Ramos, Angel, Carina Rodriguez, Paz Martinez-Beneyto, Daniel Perez, Alexandre Gault, Juan Carlos Falcon, and Patrick Boyle. 2009. 'Use of Telemedicine in the Remote Programming of Cochlear Implants.' *Acta Oto-Laryngologica* 129 (5): 533–540. doi: 10.1080/00016480802294369

Ravi, Rohit, Dhanshree R. Gunjawate, Krishna Yerraguntla, and Carlie Driscoll. 2018. 'Knowledge and Perceptions of Teleaudiology among Audiologists: A Systematic Review.' *Journal of Audiology & Otology* 22 (3): 120–127. doi: 10.7874/jao.2017.00353

Sanford, Jon A., Helen Hoenig, Patricia C. Griffiths, Tina Butterfield, Peg Richardson, and Katina Hargraves. 2007. 'A Comparison of Televideo and

Traditional In-Home Rehabilitation in Mobility Impaired Older Adults.' *Physical & Occupational Therapy in Geriatrics* 25 (3): 1–18. doi: 10.1080/J148v25n03_01

Sereda, Magdalena, Sandra Smith, Kiri Newton, and David Stockdale. 2019. 'Mobile Apps for Management of Tinnitus: Users' Survey, Quality Assessment, and Content Analysis.' *JMIR MHealth and UHealth* 7 (1): e10353. doi: 10.2196/10353

Shapiro, William H., Tina Huang, Theresa Shaw, J. Thomas Roland, and Anil K. Lalwani. 2008. 'Remote Intraoperative Monitoring during Cochlear Implant Surgery Is Feasible and Efficient.' *Otology & Neurotology* 29 (4): 495–498. doi: 10.1097/MAO.0b013e3181692838

Singh, G. 2014. 'Teleaudiology: Are Patients and Practitioners Ready for It? Stäfa.' *Phonak*, no. Switzerland. Available at: https://www.phonakpro.com/content/dam/phonakpro/gc_hq/en/events/2012/advances_in_audiology_lasvegas/Singh_G_Teleaudiology_Are_patients_and_practitioners_ready.pdf (accessed on 23 December 2019).

Singh, Gurjit, M. Kathleen Pichora-Fuller, Marissa Malkowski, Michael Boretzki, and Stefan Launer. 2014. 'A Survey of the Attitudes of Practitioners toward Teleaudiology.' *International Journal of Audiology* 53 (12): 850–860. doi: 10.3109/14992027.2014.921736

Smith, Anthony C., Karen Youngberry, Fiona Christie, Alan Isles, Robert McCrossin, Michael Williams, Jasper Van der Westhuyzen, and Richard Wootton. 2003. 'The Family Costs of Attending Hospital Outpatient Appointments via Videoconference and in Person.' *Journal of Telemedicine and Telecare* 9 (Supp. 2): S58–61. doi: 10.1258/135763303322596282

Smits, Cas, Theo S. Kapteyn, and Tammo Houtgast. 2004. 'Development and Validation of an Automatic Speech-in-Noise Screening Test by Telephone.' *International Journal of Audiology* 43 (1): 15–28.

Swanepoel, D. W. 2013. '20Q: Audiology to the People—Combining Technology and Connectivity for Services by Telehealth.' *Audiology Online* Article 12183. Available at: https://www.audiologyonline.com/articles/audiology-to-people-combining-technology-12183 (accessed on 23 December 2019).

Torsney, Kathleen. 2003. 'Advantages and Disadvantages of Telerehabilitation for Persons with Neurological Disabilities.' *NeuroRehabilitation* 18 (2): 183–185.

Victoor, Aafke, Diana MJ Delnoij, Roland D Friele, and Jany JDJM Rademakers. 2012. 'Determinants of Patient Choice of Healthcare Providers: A Scoping Review.' *BMC Health Services Research* 12 (1): 272. doi: 10.1186/1472-6963-12-272

Wesarg, Thomas, Arkadiusz Wasowski, Henryk Skarzynski, Angel Ramos, Juan Carlos Falcon Gonzalez, George Kyriafinis, FriederikeJunge, Allan Novakovich, Herbert Mauch, and Roland Laszig. 2010. 'Remote Fitting in Nucleus Cochlear Implant Recipients.' *Acta Oto-Laryngologica* 130 (12): 1379–1388. doi: 10.3109/00016489.2010.492480

Whitten, P., and B. Love. 2005. 'Patient and Provider Satisfaction with the Use of Telemedicine: Overview and Rationale for Cautious Enthusiasm.' *Journal of Postgraduate Medicine* 51: 294–300.

Whitten, Pamela S., and Michael S. Mackert. 2005. 'Addressing Telehealth's Foremost Barrier: Provider as Initial Gatekeeper.' *International Journal of Technology Assessment in Health Care* 21 (4): 517–521. doi: 10.1017/S0266462305050725

Winters, Jack M. 2002. 'Telerehabilitation Research: Emerging Opportunities.' *Annual Review of Biomedical Engineering* 4: 287–320. doi: 10.1146/annurev.bioeng.4.112801.121923

Wootton, R., and M. A. Hebert. 2001. 'What Constitutes Success in Telehealth?' *Journal of Telemedicine and Telecare* 7 (Supp. 2): 3–7. doi: 10.1258/1357633011937245

World Health Organisation. 2011. 'Telemedicine: Opportunities and Developments in Member States: Report on the Second Global Survey on Ehealth Global Observatory for Ehealth Series.' Available at: http://www.who.int/goe/publications/goe_telemedicine_2010.pdf (accessed on 23 December 2019).

Yao, Jianchu Jason, Daoyuan Yao, and Gregg Givens. 2015. 'A Browser Server Based Tele-Audiology System That Supports Multiple Hearing Test Modalities.' *Telemedicine Journal and E-Health* 21 (9): 697–704. doi: 10.1089/tmj.2014.01/1

Computer-Based Listening Training for Children with Hearing Impairment

Prashanth Prabhu P. and
Husna Firdose

Hearing impairment has a serious impact on the communicational abilities of the individuals affected with hearing loss. The prevalence of hearing loss in different age groups of the population has increased over the years and reached frightening levels. World Health Organization (WHO) has recorded 360 million (5.3% of the total population of the world) individuals in the world with hearing loss, among which, 32 million (9%) is paediatric population (WHO 2012). Also, this disabling hearing loss in the paediatric population is found to be the greatest in Asia-Pacific, Southern Asia and Sub-Saharan Africa (WHO 2012). All these reports guide us towards the importance of early identification, diagnosis and early rehabilitation. Thus there is an urge for the development of effective rehabilitation programmes to allow successful communication for all. Though there are a wide variety of communication options available for children with hearing loss, the most acceptable mode of communication is speech. Human beings express their thoughts and feelings, utilizing speech. To depend on speech, as a normal mode of communication, human beings have to depend on the sense of hearing. This creates a necessity to adequately perceive and receive speech through auditory stimuli. Thus, the sense of hearing receives a greater dependence on oral communication. The choice of communication options ranges from auditory only, visual only or a combination of both the senses along with the tactile sense, whenever appropriate. Most of the children who use appropriate amplification devices and have good aided speech perception are suited for the auditory-verbal mode of communication, but not all children. Some children might require visual cues like gestures, signs or facial expressions to understand, especially in difficult situations. Modes of communication can be broadly studied as the oral mode of communication, manual mode of communication or total communication.

Rehabilitation of children with hearing impairment is at its utmost priority to mainstream children in terms of having a normal mode of communication with their peers. Hearing impairment not only has an impact on the child's speech and language development but also hinders the child's overall social, educational and personality development. This emphasizes the need for early identification and intervention to minimize the adverse effects of hearing impairment on the holistic development of the child.

Neuroplasticity and critical age are the two important factors to be considered while discussing early identification. Neuroplasticity is the ability of the brain to change continuously throughout an individual's life. This is considered to be the main reason for prognosis due to the fact that the young child's brain is more plastic compared to an adult's brain. Thus, early identification leads to a better prognosis. The critical period is one such important factor to be considered in plasticity. The concept of the critical period was initially discussed by Lenneberg in 1967. According to Lenneberg, 'Language is biologically innate and there is an optimum time for its development. Language cannot be learnt, once this time is passed'. However, Early identification will be effective and rewarding only when it is followed by early intervention.

Although early identification and fitting of appropriate amplification devices have its importance, children must undergo proper rehabilitation programmes which include auditory therapy along with speech therapy (Bloom 2004; Boothroyd 2007, 2010; Fu and Galvin 2007; Fu et al. 2005; Martin 2007; Pallarito 2011; Sweetow and Sabes 2006). It is possible for them to develop exceptional conversational skills and academic competencies because of early identification and diagnosis of hearing loss through infant hearing screening, advances in hearing technology, medical intervention, auditory-verbal therapy, speech therapy and practice (Estabrooks 1994).

BACKGROUND

The hearing aid users in India are increasing due to the vast population of the country, coupled with more percentage of people suffering from hearing impairment. The hearing aid market is projected to increase on each successive day. A hearing aid is a man-made machine and fitting a hearing aid to a person with hearing impairment is just an initial step in the treatment for acquired hearing loss. In the next stage of the treatment, an individual with hearing impairment with a hearing aid has to undergo the training where he/she is trained to listen.

Hearing aids alone cannot lead to an improvement in the listening skills or comprehension needed for communication. As patients started realizing there are supplemental exercises available that will help them improve their listening skills through some listening activities, they started seeking these types of services. For the therapists, they must be ready to incorporate new and innovative tools into their practices. However, it is not standardized and it depends again on an individual's skills. As per the general consensus, manual auditory training has been thought to be dull and it fails in motivating the trainee if the techniques followed are monotonous and unvaried. Since there is no standardization in therapy techniques, objective measurement of the progress is not possible and also there is no reference point for any therapy technique.

Management Options Available for Children with Hearing Impairment

Post fitting of appropriate amplification devices, the rehabilitation process has expanded over the years from primitive lip-reading techniques to advanced and evidence-based techniques like auditory-verbal therapy. By and large, there are three approaches to provide auditory training: individual therapy, group therapy and also home-based therapy. Of these techniques, the home-based therapy could either be the usual one-to-one therapy or could be computer-based training. Individual therapy is more often not so feasible, taxing a lot of resources, like proper set-up, clinical expert and adequate time and usually, these services are non-reimbursable (Bloom 2004; Fitzpatrick and Brewster 2010; Pallarito 2011). This becomes a matter of concern in a country like India, where there is a lack of awareness and accessibility issues in the rural population of many states. On the contrary, group therapy can be more time and cost-efficient (Hull 2011). Nonetheless, group therapy involves a major concern for the lack of individual attention.

Introduction to Computer-Based Programmes for Rehabilitation

In this world of automation, any field for that matter has evolved itself with various technologies especially incorporating computer-based programmes for any task. This has attracted the researchers' attention wishing to develop new programmes even in this context of rehabilitation of hearing impairment individuals in terms of the development of listening skills (Bellman et al. 2011; Feijoo et al. 2012; Jain 2011). In this regard, there are several computer-based programmes designed and put forth for rehabilitating individuals with hearing impairment. The programmes which document efficacy are mostly computer-based auditory training programmes (CBATPs) concentrating on the adult population (Fu et al. 2005; Martin 2007; Oba et al. 2011; Stacey et al. 2010). Though there is a considerable number of CBATPs available in the market which could be used with children with hearing impairment, they lack efficacy measures. Oba et al. (2011) justified that the improvement noticed in the auditory performance was due to the targeted auditory training and not due to generalized improvement in memory and/or attention. Previous researchers (Pallarito 2011) have supported the notion that such research is limited. Thus, there exists a lack in the professional clinical guidelines for the use of CBATPs. A systematic review of evidence for the efficacy of individual auditory training in adults (Brouns et al. 2011; Sweetow and Palmer 2005) and children (Nanjundswamy et al. 2017) are reported in the literature.

Nanjundswamy et al. (2017) explored the fact that there exists extremely limited evidence on the efficacy of the use of these CBATPs in children with hearing impairment. According to the authors, although there exists a great deal of CBATPs commercially available to use for children with hearing impairment, the evidence on efficacy is sparse. This suggests the need for future research in establishing the efficacy of the existing programmes to be used with children with hearing impairment.

Sweetow and Palmer (2005) reported that out of 42 articles, only six articles met the criteria of their review. They highlighted that there are many articles on auditory training out of which, only a few met the precise and proper scientific criteria, like there was either lack of control groups or a small sample size, which set to qualify the evidence of their result. Thus, they concluded that the determination of the effectiveness of such programmes is essential and that more studies are required and should focus on adapting well-defined and strict criteria to be established as an evidence-based approach. Brouns et al. (2011) also reported similar methodological weaknesses and statistically significant clinically relevant outcome measures in their reviewed articles on auditory training in older adults (50 years or above) with mild to moderate sensorineural hearing loss. Along with the above shortcomings, they also suggested that the future directions of auditory training investigations should be based on the limitations in the current evidence rather than only changing and modifying the currently available techniques. Several other systematic reviews of individual CBATPs for adults with hearing impairment (Henshaw and Ferguson 2013; Pizarek et al. 2013) also describe comparable and identical research gaps that prohibit the reviewers from defining and recommending CBATPs as an evidence-based practice for adults.

Technology in today's world is not only limited to adults, but children also are in par with the adults in the use of these electronic gadgets, especially for e-learning and gaming. There exists an ocean of apps and gadgets to teach and learn the language, vocabulary building, phonetics, academic skills, etc. This is a clear indicator that children are more interested in such learning-based computer programmes. With the documented evidence of the usefulness of CBATPs with adults, the advancement of technology has led to the launch of CBATPs for children as well. However, there is a little or no documented proof of efficacy for the same. The first step in establishing the evidence and usefulness of these CBATPs for children requires a careful and precise evaluation of the currently existing programmes, their content and the structure. In turn, this would help researchers to identify and fill in the gaps and fields that require modifications and improvements in the currently available programmes and consequently bring about more and more research aiming at establishing and developing evidence-based practices (Brouns et al. 2011) in CBATPs, especially for the paediatric population. Such results retrieved with randomized controlled trials will assist scientific learning and comprehending whether CBATPs can be of any assistance to individuals with hearing impairment. Yet, such scientific awareness is mostly derived from the primitive level of expert opinions, case series, clinical experience or the case reports.

MAIN FOCUS OF THE CHAPTER

To precisely investigate the currently available CBATPs developed for children with hearing impairment and also the documentation of their effectiveness, if any. This chapter will refresh and renew the clinicians and the researchers' knowledge on the training programmes that can profitably be used for paediatric population with hearing impairment. It will also empower the possessors of the currently available programmes to record relevant efficacy measures and assist the forthcoming researches to competently fill the voids by establishing well-designed programmes with suitable efficacy results and measures.

Success of CBATPs

Nanjundaswamy et al. (2017) critically reviewed research articles carried out in the area of CBATPs and had concluded the existence of a lack of research on children using CBATPs. Out of abstracts of 124 articles, 120 were rejected based on the inclusion and exclusion criteria. Although there is a lack of efficacy measurements, there exist many commercially available CBATPs that have a lot of activities and concepts available for various age groups.

A careful and comprehensive study was carried out on the efficacy of LiSN and Learn auditory training software in the children and the adults with hearing impairment by Glyde, Sharon, Harvey and Louis (2014). Keeping in mind that the changes at the peripheral level (like distortions of interaural level and time differences, before they leave the cochlea and not from the deficits at higher levels) (Cameron and Dillon 2011) results in the deficits in the spatial processing in individuals with hearing impairment. The efficacy of the software in the population with hearing impairment was also studied. The researchers concluded that there was no significant difference in the spacial processing of an individual with hearing impairment due to training. Also, no significant difference was seen between the two groups, but the reasons for the same are stated in an unclear manner.

Available CBATPs for Individuals with Hearing Impairment

Although there are several CBATPs, there is scarcity in the research providing the efficacy of these programmes. Some of these commercially available programmes are listed below. These programmes are specially designed for the paediatric population affected with hearing impairment. They include Angel Sound Training (TigerSpeech Technology, Hefei, China), programmes offered by Cochlear (Sydney, Australia), programmes offered by MED-EL (Innsbruck, Austria), Otto's World of Sounds (Oticon, Somerset, NJ, US), programmes offered by Advanced Bionics (Valencia, CA, US), home auditory training programme (HAP) and computerized auditory training for Kannada speaking children with hearing impairment (CAT for KASHI).

Tiger Speech technology developed a programme named Angel Sound Training which was distributed by the Emily Shannon Fu Foundation. This is an interactive computer-based programme for auditory training and hearing assessment. It has a PC-based rehabilitation programme as well as a mobile version which assists the parents and the caregivers in supplementing professional rehabilitation programme at home as well. This auditory rehabilitation programme is potentially self-administrable. This programme includes a vast range of activities and stimulus including non-verbal stimuli to a verbal stimulus like syllables, words and sentences. There are nine modules, including stimulus, both in quiet environment and in the presence of noise. Each of these modules has various levels of difficulties. Other activities like music and cognition are also included.

Practice on discrimination and also identification of sounds and speech components is possible via a series of modules covering different aspects of the listening process. These modules are self-paced and the difficulty level can be manipulated according to the child's listening behaviour. Audio-Visual feedback is also provided. It can be freely downloaded from the Internet. This programme is comprehensible and it is bounded in terms of the concepts that the modules cover.

The mobile division of Tiger Speech Technology Inc. and Emily Fu Foundation is developed by Inconvenient Solutions, called as the i-Angel Sound. This is dedicated to expanding innovative speech software for children with hearing impairment in facilitating the learning of sounds. It includes a few thousand sounds from various categories, including the names of the common foods, environmental sounds, monosyllabic words and the name of familiar animals. The monosyllabic word training uses a phonetic contrast training protocols which reinforce the brain's ability to distinguish between phonemes. These phonemes are considered as the building blocks of language. This programme gives an opportunity to everyone who enjoys listening to different environmental sounds and music and it can also improve the speech perception in any individual.

Sound Explorer is a simplified mobile edition of Angel Sound programme. This has its application in auditory training as well as hearing assessment. Along with the aforementioned modules, it also includes several other programmes to improve various higher-level auditory skills. To work on working memory, a digit memory span test is included. To assess and improve speech perception in noise in older children with hearing impairment, a digit in noise test is included. Concatenated sentence recognition in noise test is to assess and also to further train the older children's ability to identify sentences in the background noise using a closed-set approach. Last but not the least, in order to improve music appreciation, the training programme includes a unique 'melodic contour identification' testing and training.

Another multimedia auditory training tool developed by Oticon is termed as Otto's World of Sounds. The basis for this module is training software in French called La Souris Bleue (The Blue Mouse) which was introduced in 1999 by Alain Vinet, a French audiologist, along with Denis Barbier, a computer scientist by profession (Carey 2006). It aims at assisting the parents and the caregivers of the children with hearing impairment to provide auditory training at home and supplement training given by professionals. It is a game-based programme which runs on a PC. Children in the age range of below than eight years avail this module for free of cost with hearing aids procured from Oticon. This programme is designed to improve auditory skills including detecting, discriminating and identifying sounds in children with hearing impairment of the age range of two and a half years to eight years. The programme runs through a CD-ROM. It includes numerous interactive and interesting activities which require the caretaker's participation in terms of assisting the child. This programme includes 10 different and distinct auditory environments, each focusing on 10 distinct sounds. A child's everyday environment is considered and sounds are selected for sound detection, sound discrimination and also sound identification. It also includes activities for discovery, memory and recognition, within each of these environments. And this follows a hierarchy. Along with the aforementioned auditory skills, the concept of vocabulary building is also focused. There are supporting training booklets also available like; Otto Hears many things, Otto's Exercise book and also Otto discovers FM.

Carey (2006) investigated the effects of Otto's world of sound on speech perception, auditory discrimination and auditory attention skills in children with hearing impairment. Four school-age children, diagnosed with moderate to profound hearing impairment, were recruited for the study. Pre- and post-training skills were compared. The results were promising for auditory attention skills and speech perception skills. But further research is warranted to demonstrate the efficacy of the training using the current software, using a randomized control study with a larger group of participants.

As in any other field of science, there is tremendous growth in the use of mobile applications in the field of rehabilitative audiology as well. These mobile apps aim at providing effective and low-cost health service delivery. With the increasing number and ease of use of the mobile phone by the general public, technologists in the field of audiology also are striving hard to create innovative and advanced apps to be used for rehabilitating children with hearing loss aiming to improve the service delivery.

Advanced Bionics (AB), one of the cochlear implant company, has also developed various rehabilitation-based programmes for both adults and children. AB Listening Adventures and VocAB Scenes could be used for children. For children aged between four and 10 years, AB Listening Adventures is best suited. It is an interactive app which provides children with hearing impairment with an interesting way to practice listening for different words in sentences. This is intended to guide the parents/caregivers or the therapists to develop language and listening skills in children with hearing impairment. Six various story-based games which target on listening to words in sentences are used to guide language development and listening skills in children. These story-based games target on improving listening skills for plurals, multiple elements, minimal pairs or pronouns. Including greater than 100 sets of words, it provides various opportunities to teach sentence structure and also build vocabulary.

For children in the age range of four and 10 years, VocAB Scenes is also one of the best suited app. It is a fun-based entertaining and colourful app to teach common vocabulary and question forms through listening. The parents/caregivers and also the therapist play an important role in developing these skills in children. A child's environment is utilized to expand vocabulary. There are six different scenes and three different games for each scene. Outside water fun, beach, pet store, swimming pool, camping, and water fun are the scenes included. Also, there are a variety of 12 drag and drop items available for each scene. This is a vocabulary-building app based on scenes. Overall, it is intended to promote language development and listening skills in children with hearing impairment.

MED-EL, a cochlear implant company, has also introduced various rehabilitation programmes for both the adults and the children. One among them is freely downloadable from the company's website called Sound Scape. This module has eight modules, and among which, only the first six can be used for children. This follows a hierarchy for various age groups from zero to two-plus years till teenage. The module called Starting Out is for children in the age range of zero to two-plus years; Ms. Mac Donald's Shed for two-plus years; Old MacDonald's Farm for two-plus years; Let's Go Shopping for six-plus years; Telling Tales for ten plus years and Continents & Oceans for the teens. There are sublevels within each module. Different activities with a hierarchy of levels of difficulty are covered which involve age-appropriate stimuli including words and phrases to sentences and paragraphs. The above-mentioned programmes also include various levels of additional activities with different difficulty levels which can be downloaded for free from the website.

Another cochlear implant company called Cochlear also provides rehabilitation programmes for users of all ages. Kaci's games and HOPE Words are a few of the programmes for children. Alphabets-based activities are used to focus on basic vocabulary building and phonetics using a preliminary app called HOPE Words. It is an auditory rehabilitation app for iPad and iPhone. This app has been manufactured as a tool to improve listening and spoken language skills in children with hearing impairment. It has been adopted from Speech sounds vowels and Speech sounds, which are two well-known HOPE resources with an intention to expose children to the speech sounds in English language. It includes interesting flashcards for all the speech sounds. Each letter of the alphabet in English has 20 different flashcards. The app includes four HOPE resources for spoken language and also for listening. They are,

- Speech sounds
- Speech sounds vowels
- Hope tips: Learning with literacy
- HOPE bulletin: Vocabulary development for children with cochlear implants

Kaci's games, another programme by Cochlear, is all about remembering matching objects. It includes two fun and interactive games to work on the same. Sounds corresponding to animal pictures are shown using various cards.

Efficacy of CBATPs in India

Apart from the above-mentioned training programmes, there are a couple of studies on the efficacy of training software in Indian languages. Kant and Adhyaru (2009) developed a kit in Marathi and Hindi languages including audio cassettes and CD-ROMs to enable teachers, caregivers and parents of the children with hearing impairment to improve auditory skills. The final content include audiocassettes, worksheets and CD-ROMs.

Materials were prepared based on the survey of CD-ROMs, audio cassettes and also nursery rhymes presently available in the market. The developed materials were tested on children with hearing impairment using cochlear implants and also hearing aids. Questionnaires were administered on the parents and the teachers of the special schools to get feedback on stimuli used and activities for auditory training. The study included a variety of environmental sounds in various contexts. The environmental sounds were embedded in poems which is a more natural and acceptable learning method.

Similarly, the stimulus for the other levels of auditory training was systematically and scientifically selected. Based on surveys and taking into consideration the parental perspective on their experience with normal-hearing children, the stimulus was further recorded. A booklet of stimulus, wherever appropriate, was made using pictures of the sound stimuli and visuals of stimulus context. Professionals and appropriate technicians and technologists participated and worked wherever they found it appropriate.

Two groups of children were recruited for the study. Different groups of children were included for different levels of auditory training. One group was the control group and the other was an experimental group. The children were provisionally diagnosed as having bilateral severe or profound sensorineural hearing loss. They were using appropriate amplification devices. Field testing was done on all the levels of auditory training. Validation of test materials was performed. Power of discrimination of each stimulus was done.

The following were the phases of the study included:

- Field testing of the developed material
- Pre-training
- Training on different auditory skills, including auditory awareness, auditory discrimination, suprasegmental perception, and identification and also auditory comprehension
- Demonstration to the parents
- Five sessions of training

Feedback from the professionals and the parents was used to comment on the effectiveness of the training stimuli and the activities. At every level of auditory training, a paired t-test was carried out to compare the responses of the pre-training and post-training phases. A significant improvement ($p < 0.05$), was observed for all the sounds except a few sounds. Parents reported that the activities were helpful to teach. The activities were easy which attracted the child's attention. Finally, the materials were field-tested in five special schools for children with hearing impairment of the state. They obtained a positive response from the parents, the teachers and the school children.

Nanjundaswamy et al. (2017) focused on evaluating the benefits of a computerized auditory training software for Kannada speaking children with a hearing impairment which concentrated on the parents' perspectives for the same. The software (Computerized Auditory training for Kannada Speaking children with Hearing Impairment-CAT for KASHI) was developed and was administered on children with hearing impairment whose mother tongue was Kannada. Few of the practical aspects of auditory rehabilitation of children with hearing impairment were taken care of. It covered activities on auditory awareness, auditory discrimination, auditory identification, auditory memory and sequencing and auditory comprehension. Questionnaires were used to check the efficacy of the software which showed improvement in the scores suggesting that software was an effective tool for training children with hearing impairment. As reported by the authors, there was positive feedback from the parents indicating a new start for the utility of the software for auditory rehabilitation of the children with hearing impairment.

Thus, to conclude, technologists in the field of auditory rehabilitation for children with hearing impairment are on par with any other health sciences. As discussed in this chapter, there are a great number of commercially available programmes to be used with children with hearing impairment. Thus to make such advances in technologies in rehabilitating these children valuable and worthwhile, evidence for the efficacy of these programmes requires immediate demand.

Benefits and Limitations of CBATPs

In today's world, CBATPs assist professionals in the field of rehabilitation to be in par with the latest technology. Since most of the available programmes are free, these programmes become affordable and convenient to be used. They can be accessed by the parents in providing at-home training which leads to a better prognosis. These techniques can be easily programmed to objectively measure and evaluate the prognosis, which is one of the major aspects of any rehabilitation programme. There is always room to update and improvise such software packages and programmes, in terms of techniques and activities, as per the requirement and need of the therapist. Such programmes can be tailor-made to be used with children with hearing loss at a different level of auditory development. However, there are also limitations for using such programmes. As discussed in this chapter, determining efficacy is a major and primary concern to use such programmes effectively and confidently. Efficacy studies of such programmes are currently lacking. Language is another major concern to use such programmes. The materials and activities should be available in the child's primary language. Parental support and parental education are a crucial factor for better or poor prognosis, when such programmes are to be used for home training and home training is a vital advantage of these CBATPs. The therapist should carefully examine and evaluate the benefits and limitations of these CBATPs before implementing their rehabilitation process.

FUTURE DIRECTIONS

This chapter will direct researchers to develop training programmes that can profitably be used for paediatric population with hearing impairment. These programmes can be developed in various regional languages considering India as a unique country which has a legacy of the diversity of languages. This will further lead to the development, improvement and standardization of the various methods and test materials suitable for auditory training to the children with hearing impairment.

Studies on the efficacy of these training programmes must be focused leading to better evidence-based training programmes for children with hearing impairment. In a multilingual country like India, there is a need to develop language-specific and systematic auditory training programmes. Thus, a new beginning towards the implementation of these CBATPs with evidence that such training programmes would benefit children with hearing impairment can be dreamt of.

CONCLUSION

The current chapter aimed to evaluate the efficacy of a computer-based auditory training programme in children with hearing impairment. In today's world, where technology has become a part of human life and one cannot imagine life without electronic devices and gadgets, professionals in the field of rehabilitation have to utilize certain aspects of these technological developments. Latest generation Cochlear implants and hearing aid technology has received a boon from the advances in computer technology. These advances ultimately benefit children using these devices by utilizing rehabilitation tools which have evolved secondarily to the development of such technology. Proper tools, resources and also, motivation will lead to a successful outcome in rehabilitation.

One such aspect of the evolution of technology into rehabilitation field is the Computer Based Auditory Training Programmes (CBATPs) for rehabilitating both adults and children with hearing impairment. Researchers have put in a great effort in developing these CBATPs in auditory training. Previous literature has consistently documented significant improvements in music and speech perception with moderate amounts of computer-based training which also provides audio-visual feedback in adult population with hearing impairment. Though there are several CBATPs available for children as well, there is a scarcity in the research providing the efficacy of these programmes. One can justify the utility of such CBATPs only based on evidence-based research suggesting the efficacy of such programmes.

The chapter tried to precisely investigate the currently available CBATPs developed for children with hearing impairment and also attempted to document their effectiveness, if any. There exist many commercially available CBATPs that include a lot of activities and concepts available for various age groups, but they lack in efficacy measurements. The chapter was focused on the following programmes. The basis was in terms of the stimulus utilized, activities and modules covered, potential candidates in terms of the age, etc. They include, Angel Sound Training (TigerSpeech Technology, Hefei, China), programmes offered by Cochlear (Sydney, Australia), programmes offered by MED-EL (Innsbruck, Austria), Otto's World of Sounds (Oticon, Somerset, NJ, US), programmes offered by Advanced Bionics (Valencia, CA, US), Home auditory training programme (HAP) and Computerized Auditory training for Kannada Speaking children with Hearing Impairment (CAT for KASHI).

REFERENCES

Bellman, Steven., Potter Robert F., Treleaven-Hassard Shiree, Robinson Jennifer A., and Varan Duane. 2011, November. 'The Effectiveness of Branded Mobile Phone Apps.' *Journal of Interactive Marketing* 2 (4): 191–200.

Bloom, Sara. 2004, August. 'Technologic Advances Raise Prospects for a Resurgence in Use of Auditory Training.' *Hear* 57 (8):19–20, 22–24.

Boothroyd, Arthur. 2007, June. 'Adult Aural Rehabilitation: What Is It and Does It Work?.' *Trends in Amplification* 11 (2): 63–71.

Boothroyd, Arthur. 2010, October. 'Adapting to Changed Hearing: The Potential Role of Formal Training.' *Journal of American Academy of Audiology* 21 (9): 601–611.

Brouns, Kit, Refaie Amr El El, and Pryce Helen. 2011, April. 'Auditory Training and Adult Rehabilitation: A Critical Review of the Evidence.' *Global journal of health science* 3 (1): 49–63.

Cameron, Sharon., and Harvey Dillon. 2011, November–December. 'Development and Evaluation of the LiSN & Learn Auditory Training Software for Deficit-specific Remediation of Binaural Processing Deficits in Children: Preliminary Findings.' *Journal of American Academy of Audiology* 22 (10): 678–696.

Carey, Anna. 2006. 'The Effectiveness of Otto's World of Sound Computer-Based Auditory Training for Improving Auditory Discrimination and Auditory Attention Skills in Children Who Have a Hearing Impairment.' ResearchSpace@ Auckland. Available at: https://researchspace.auckland.ac.nz/handle/2292/405 (accessed on 24 December 2019).

Estabrooks, Warren., ed. 1994. *Auditory–Verbal Therapy: For Parents and Professionals.* Washington, DC: Alexander Graham Bell Association for the Deaf.

Feijoo, Claudio, Gómez-Barroso José-Luis, Aguado Juan-Miguel, and Ramos Sergio. 2012, April. 'Mobile Gaming: Industry Challenges and Policy Implications.' *Telecommunications Policy* 36, (3): 212–221.

Fitzpatrick Elizabeth M., and Brewster Lynnes. 2010. 'Adult cochlear implantation in Canada: Results of a survey.' *Canadian Journal* of *Speech-Language Pathology* and *Audiology* 34 (4): 290–296.

Fu, Qian-Jie, and John J. Galvin. 2005, June. 'Auditory Training with Spectrally Shifted Speech: Implications for Cochlear Implant Patient Auditory Rehabilitation.' *Journal of Association for Research in Otolaryngology* 6 (2): 180–189.

Fu, Qian-Jie, and John J. Galvin. 2007, September. 'Perceptual Learning and Auditory Training in Cochlear Implant Recipients.' *Trends in Amplification* 11 (3): 193–205.

Glyde Helen, Cameron Sharon, Dillon Harvey, and Hickson Louise. 2014, June. 'Remediation of Spatial Processing Deficits in Hearing-Impaired Children and Adults'. *Journal of American Academy of Audiology* 25 (6): 549–561.

Helen Henshaw and Ferguson Melanie A. 2013, May. 'Efficacy of Individual Computer-based Auditory Training for People with Hearing Loss: A Systematic Review of the Evidence.' *PLOS ONE* 8 (5): e62836.

Hull, Raymond H. 2011, April. 'A Brief Treatise on the Service of Aural Rehabilitation.' *Hearing Journal* 64 (4): 14, 16, 18.

Jain, Ashish. 2011, August. 'Apps market places and the telecom value chain.' *IEEE Wireless Communications* 18 (4): 4–5.

Kant, Anjali, and Adhyaru, Medha. 2009, March. 'Home Auditory Training Program (HAP) for Cochlear Implantees and Hearing Impaired Children Using Hearing Aids-An Outcome of a Three-Year Research Project.' *Indian Journal of Otolaryngology and Head and Neck Surgery* 61 (1): 54–58.

Lenneberg, Eric H. 1967. 'The Biological Foundations of Language.' *Hospital Practice* 2 (12): 59–67.

Martin, Melody. 2007, August. 'Software-based Auditory Training Program Found to Reduce Hearing Aid Return Rate.' *Hearing Journal* 60 (8): 32–35.

Nanjundaswamy Manohar, Prabhu Prashanth, Rajanna Revathi K., Ningegowda Raghavendra G., Firdose Husna, and Sharma Madhuri. 2017, October. 'Benefits of Computerized Auditory Training Software for Kannada Speaking Children with Hearing Impairment—Parent's Perspective.' *Hearing, Balance and Communication* 15 (4): 227–234.

Oba Sandra I., Fu Qian-Jie, and Galvin John J. 2011, September–October. 'Digit Training in Noise Can Improve Cochlear Implant Users' Speech Understanding in Noise.' *Ear and Hearing* 32 (5): 573–581.

Pallarito, Karen. 2011. 'Retraining the Brain When Hearing Aids Are Not Enough.' *Hearing Journal*, 64 (8): 25, 26, 30, 31, 32, 34.

Pizarek Rachel, Shafiro Valeriy, and McCarthy Patricia. 2013, December. 'Effect of Computerized Auditory Training on Speech Perception of Adults with Hearing Impairment.' *Perspectives on Aural Rehabilitation and Its Instrumentation* 20 (3): 91.

Stacey Paula C., Raine Christopher H., O'Donoghue Gerard M., Tapper Lynne, Twomey Tracey, and Summerfield A. Quentin. 2010, April. 'Effectiveness of Computer-based Auditory Training for Adult Users of Cochlear Implants.' *International Journal of Audiology* 49 (5): 347–356

Sweetow, Robert W., and Sabes Jennifer H. 2006, September. 'The Need for and Development of an Adaptive Listening and Communication Enhancement (LACE) Program.' *Journal of American Academy of Audiology* 17 (8): 538–558.

Sweetow Robert, and Palmer Catherine V. 2005, July–August. 'Efficacy of Individual Auditory Training in Adults: A Systematic Review of the Evidence.' *Journal of American Academy of Audiology* 16 (7): 494–504.

WHO. 2012. *WHO Global Estimates on Prevalence of Hearing Loss*. Geneva: World Health Organization. Available at: http://www.who.int/pbd/deafness/estimates (accessed on 24 December 2019).

Web- or App-Based Assessment and Management of Tinnitus

Prashanth Prabhu P. and Megha K. N.

INTRODUCTION

Tinnitus is characterized by the perception of sound without an existing external stimulus (Henry, Dennis and Schechter 2005). The presence of tinnitus might be intolerable for many and could be sufficiently troublesome in hearing, sleeping, thought processing and other functional abilities, all of which can negatively impact the quality of life (Henry, Dennis and Schechter 2005; Nondahl et al. 2007). Tinnitus can be classified into three major types. The first type is objective tinnitus, which is caused by sounds generated somewhere in the body, for example, turbulent flow of blood or muscle contractions in the head, which can be heard externally. The second type is subjective tinnitus, which is the perception of meaningless sounds without any actual physical sound present. The last type is auditory hallucinations, which are perceptions of meaningful sounds, such as music or speech. The latter two types are phantom sensations (Jastreboff, 1990, 1995). The authors are focusing more on subjective tinnitus in this chapter which is the most prevalent type and can be of varying severity. Subjective tinnitus can sound very subtle to very disturbing sounds, like a continuous roar. A severe form of tinnitus is frequently associated with other symptoms like hyperacusis or sound distortion. Other disorders like depression and phonophobia, often accompany tinnitus and sometimes can lead to suicide (Møller 2003). For reasons unstated, about 20 per cent of the individuals who experience tinnitus account that it negatively affects their lives to the extent that clinical intervention is necessary (Davis and El Refaie, 2000; Jastreboff, Hazell and Vernon, 1998).

Epidemiologic studies have reported tinnitus as a common problem for millions of people with its prevalence ranging between 8 per cent and 25.3 per cent of the population in the United States (Adams, Hendershot and Marano 1999; KochKin, Tyler and Born 2011; Nondahl et al. 2002, 2011; Shargorodsky, Curhan and Farwell 2010). Many population-based studies conducted in other nations have found similar results wherein, the prevalence of tinnitus ranges from 4.6 per cent to 30 per cent (Jalessi et al. 2013; Khedr et al. 2010; Park and Moon 2014; Quaranta, Assennato; Sallustio 1996, and Sindhusake et al. 2003). In the general population, approximately 10–15 per cent are affected by tinnitus, whereas 70–90 per cent of the patients attending the otology clinic experience tinnitus either as an associated symptom or as the main complaint. The single most important factor affecting the prevalence of tinnitus is hearing impairment and the associated increase in risk is dependent on the severity of hearing impairment (Heller 2003; Nondahl et al. 2011, 2002; Shargorodsky, Curhan and Farwell 2010). The lack of objective signs and inadequate understanding of the pathology of tinnitus are the problems innately present in the treatment of tinnitus. Having such differences in attributes, it is not rational to possibly think of a single cause or mechanism causing tinnitus. Likewise, many studies have highlighted various causes for the generation of tinnitus. Evidence from most of the studies states that there could be a central mechanism involved in the production of tinnitus. Few of the models which proposed this include spontaneous activity in the neural system in the absence of external stimuli. An argument to support this view was the destruction of cochlear function, specifically the inner hair cells destroy spontaneous activity of auditory nerve fibres whereas, there is no effect when there is an outer hair cell damage suggesting that the activity is more pronounced at the peripheral level and commonly attributed to stochastic spontaneous transmitter release from receptor cells (Dallos and Harris 1978). Other theories associated with the neuronal system include increased burst firing, pathological synchronization of neural activity, hypersensitivity and reorganization (Eggermont 1990; Martin 1995; Ochi and

Eggermont 1996). Similarly, discordant damage of inner & outer hair cells, spontaneous otoacoustic emissions were proposed for explaining the generation of tinnitus at the cochlear level (Jastreboff, 1990, 1995; Stypulkowski, 1990).

A routine audiological evaluation including pure-tone audiometry, speech audiometry, immittance measures and otoacoustic emissions would be carried out but is of less usefulness in finding the characteristics of tinnitus. However, these evaluations are important to find out whether tinnitus is associated with conductive pathology, cochlear or retro-cochlear pathology for management. The traditional approach to assess the tinnitus characteristics would be pitch matching, loudness matching and to determine whether the residual inhibition was positive (where the tinnitus is not perceived after the presentation of white noise), negative (where there is no effect on tinnitus loudness after presentation of noise) or partially positive (where there is incomplete/partial recovery from tinnitus, however, it persists). Besides these being important tests in evaluating the characteristics of tinnitus, many studies have reported a weak relation of the findings from these tests and to the self-reported tinnitus levels (Jakes, Hallam, Rachman and Hinchcliffe, 1986; Jakes, Hallam, Chambers and Hinchcliffe, 1985; Meikle and Taylor-Walsh, 1984).

It is evident that for many individuals with chronic tinnitus, intervention is not required. Having said that, the severity of symptoms may be tolerable. The most frequently discussed intervention for the management of tinnitus was medical treatment, although it is not recommended (Bhatt, Lin and Bhattacharyya 2016). The recommendation against medical therapy is principally due to inadequate evidence to reveal a decline in the perception of tinnitus from experimental trials and meta-analyses (Tunkel et al. 2014). Few of the commonly used treatment procedures for tinnitus include sound amplification/sound generators (Tunkel et al. 2014); Tinnitus retraining therapy (Wu et al. 2018); and, cognitive behavioural therapy (Jun and Park 2013). In recent years, there has been a growing interest in the Internet- and smartphone-based technologies for the management of individuals with tinnitus. There is a broad spectrum of approaches relevant in the treatment of tinnitus, which could be through experimental studies or through products that are marketed, reported in the literature.

They include questionnaires, auditory treatments, Internet-based Cognitive Behavioural Therapy (iCBT; Kalle et al. 2018) and games present in different operating systems including web/Android/iOS for tinnitus monitoring and management. The goal of this chapter is to underline the role of existing web or app-based applications for the betterment of tinnitus-related problems.

Background

The preliminary assessment procedure for tinnitus includes recording case history which helps in differential diagnosis. The most important history details which would help in this aspect include exposure to occupational noise, if under any medication (ototoxic) and acoustic trauma. Other general aspects that are essential include asking about the type of tinnitus that is, low pitched or high pitched, pulsatile or continuous, unilateral or bilateral. Associated symptoms, like hearing loss and vertigo, are counted upon for focal neurologic symptoms. The next step in assessment is physical examination which could be directed based on the history. Because tinnitus can have various origins, the physical examination is symptom-based. The examinations include looking for signs of ear infection, tympanic membrane perforation, tumours, neck examination and cranial nerve examination. Further, audiological evaluations are performed to help determine the degree of hearing loss, if present, and to know how tinnitus is perceived (Henry, Dennis and Schechter 2005; Tunkel et al. 2014). As a whole, tinnitus evaluation in practice includes pitch matching, loudness matching, maskability and residual inhibition (Henry et al. 2004). However, an in-depth assessment would vary from the type and severity of tinnitus. This includes imaging tests, most often for individuals with unilateral tinnitus as well as pulsatile tinnitus; for bilateral tinnitus and non-pulsatile unilateral tinnitus having asymmetrical sensory-neural hearing loss a referral to an otolaryngologist is recommended (Fortnum et al. 2009). Apart from these evaluations, Internet-based assessment procedures are also available. This mode of assessment is mainly applicable for individuals who are isolated from the mainland or who cannot access the facility due to their immobility. Track Your Tinnitus is one such application available with good efficacy rates and others include Tinnitus Clinic Information, Hearing screen or assessment of ambient sound levels.

In terms of management of tinnitus, sound amplification can be used as it is usually associated with sensorineural hearing loss (Portnuff 2016). However, many individuals report of tinnitus without any complaints in hearing sensitivity (Barnea et al. 2009; Gu et al. 2010) with whom sound amplification is not the line of treatment. Conservative management can be used in them to relieve the symptoms of tinnitus and also to improve the Quality of Life (QOL) by helping in improving sleep, reducing stress and anxiety (Folmer, Martin and Shi 2004). Sound amplification will also help some individuals with tinnitus to find relief which operates as a masker by introducing ambient noise. Also, specialized tinnitus maskers and white noise generators are available which provide adjustable sounds or different noise types for additional assistance (Hazell and Wood 1981; Sandlin and Olsson 1999; Tunkel et al. 2014). The most commonly used rehabilitation therapy for treating tinnitus is tinnitus retraining therapy which plays a key role in disassociating patient's negative emotions to tinnitus by directive counselling and sound therapy (Wu et al. 2018); and, cognitive behavioural therapy (CBT) which focuses on counselling and relaxation therapy (Jun and Park 2013). An Internet-based CBT (iCBT) has also came to existence for treating tinnitus. In the past, there has been an increasing trend in using smartphone-based/Internet-based applications in helping individuals with tinnitus to recover. These apps may offer various therapy sounds useful in tinnitus relief. Some of these apps also contain added relaxation and sleep techniques for tinnitus management. To name a few of these applications: Resound Relief, Beltone Tinnitus Calmer, Track your tinnitus and so on. The information on different applications will be discussed in detail.

WEB/ANDROID/IOS-BASED APPLICATIONS IN ASSESSMENT AND MANAGEMENT OF TINNITUS

Tinnitus is a condition that can have different origins; hence, the use of different treatment methods and the improvement from these treatments can also vary. Psychological interventions, like CBT, at present have a good amount of evidence of efficacy in reducing tinnitus-related distress (Cima et al. 2014; Hesser et al. 2011). Despite having good efficacy in reducing tinnitus distress, it is rarely offered in clinical practice due to shortage of service delivering professionals, especially in remote areas and associated costs (Andersson 2015; Gander et al. 2011; Hoare et al. 2011). As more people access the Internet in recent, it is more accepted and is more often used by patients to access information on health care (Eysenbach et al. 1998). It is possible that the Internet can change the mode of providing health care in the future and hence there is a need to assess the advantages and the disadvantages of Internet administrated treatment. One of the most advanced and popular approaches in treating tinnitus through the Internet are iCBT. In particular, CBT was initially developed and evaluated with anxiety and affective disorders (Hawton et al. 1989). This has been established to provide coping strategies and relief for individuals with tinnitus (Andersson et al. 1995). Numerous studies have reviewed and presented a positive outcome via iCBT, that is, individuals with tinnitus have reported a reduction in anxiety, distress related to tinnitus, stress, annoyance and an improvement in the QOL (Andersson 2015; Andersson et al. 2002, 2014).

ASSESSMENT OF TINNITUS

Assessment procedures encompass the use of questionnaires in order to collect patient assessments and further information and also, for other diagnostic procedures like tinnitus matching. The diagnostic or assessment procedures are very often linked to tinnitus treatment (Kalle et al. 2018).

Due to the heterogeneity of this condition and the fact that tinnitus is a fluctuating condition, so far there is no management option available that can help reduce tinnitus reliably. A better way to assess tinnitus is by conducting longitudinal measurements which are difficult to achieve using traditional research methods like clinical interviews and paper-and-pencil questionnaires (Schlee et al. 2016). Modern technologies have helped in gaining access to subjective measurement under real-life conditions with the help of portable electronic devices which in turn helps in collecting longitudinal data. Ecological momentary assessment (EMA) is one such concept that is being used for real-life subjective measurements for more reliable assessment. However, recently smartphone applications have taken over portable devices adding to the lesser cost. Track Your Tinnitus (TYT) is an application compatible with both iOS and Android devices. TYT is an open-access platform at no costs for the users. It was developed by the Tinnitus Research Initiative (TRI) and the Institute for Databases and Information Systems (DBIS) at the University of Ulm. A detailed description of the technical aspects is published elsewhere (Pryss, Reichert, Herrmann et al. 2015; Pryss, Reichert, Langguth et al. 2015; Schickler et al. 2015). The TYT mainly focuses on two aspects namely 'tinnitus loudness' and 'tinnitus distresses'. Recent studies have shown to have no significant negative effects of both distress and loudness after using this application (Schlee et al. 2016) and concluded that TYT could be recommended for everyday monitoring of tinnitus.

Another development in the field of tinnitus assessment was a 'mobile serious game' which focused on suppressing irrelevant (tinnitus) background sounds and focus on target sound. A concept called Audio Defence was incorporated in this game wherein, individuals are presented sounds having different sources and directions without visual information. The participants are instructed to fight the opponents by relying on the acoustic stimuli by determining the direction of the opponent sounds generated by an audio defence. Schickler et al. (2016) reported that this game is feasible for individuals affected by tinnitus which helps in suppressing tinnitus by focusing on directional hearing. The advantages listed in the same study were its all-time availability, feedback to the players, individuals enjoying the game and hence, improved motivation; and finally a hierarchical difficulty level. There are many applications available in Google Play Store, to name a few, Tinnitus Tester 2, 3 and 4, Tinnitus Describer, Tinnitus symptoms, and Treatment, Hearing screen or assessment of ambient sound levels. However, no studies have indicated the efficacy of the usage of these applications.

MANAGEMENT OF TINNITUS

Treatment of tinnitus is a broad area that talks about both psychological as well as auditory-based treatment. Psychological treatment would mainly focus on CBT which has been reviewed and has been reported to have good efficacy in treating tinnitus. In addition, Acceptance and Commitment Therapy (ACT) has also been used as a self-help format using Internet mode for treating tinnitus (Westin et al. 2011). Studies comparing iCBT and ACT have concluded that both these treatment methods have resulted in similar improvement in tinnitus distress (Hesser et al. 2012). Auditory treatment for tinnitus includes tinnitus maskers, environmental sound generators, hearing aids and a combination of the above-mentioned devices based on individual needs (Kalle et al. 2018). The focus of iCBT and ACT is described in brief below.

Internet-Based Cognitive Behavioural Therapy (iCBT)

Internet-delivered cognitive behaviour therapy is considered to have the best evidence from the literature of the various counselling methods (Martinez-Devesa et al. 2010; Westin, Hayes and Andersson 2008). Treatment using iCBT mainly emphasizes reframing the perception of incidents (e.g., tinnitus) by an individual which further helps in assisting shift in attention and enhances the sense of control (Andersson and Mckenna 2006). Interventions assisted through Internet delivery have many advantages over the traditional forms of treatment. The major advantages include: saving the time of the therapists, patients get their own space during assessment and therapy procedures, which further help them to have a more fair opinion about their problem, minimizing waiting-lists, cutting down travelling time and expenses, reducing the stigma for people living in rural or remote areas (Marks, Cavanagh and Gega 2007). However, there are few disadvantages too, such as not being feasible for individuals with no or limited education, not being able to ask all the questions and misunderstanding by the patients (Marks, Cavanagh and Gega 2007).

Acceptance and Commitment Therapy (ACT)

The ACT has been considered as one of the alternatives for CBT which helps in permitting a link between emotional, cognitive and physical sensations without altering their general functioning (Hesser et al. 2012; Westin, Hayes and Andersson 2008). The concept of acceptance has been highlighted in many of the previous studies as a supporting method for the treatment of tinnitus (Tyler, Coelho and Noble 2006). There is correlational and experimental data which shows that acceptance is related to better functioning and well-being in chronic pain (Vowles, McCracken and Eccleston 2007; McCracken 1998). Outcome studies have shown promising results of ACT for patients with chronic pain (Vowles and McCracken 2008; Wicksell et al. 2009). Hence, it has been proven that ACT is an alternative treatment approach for the treatment of tinnitus.

Tinnitus relief apps provide different types of therapy sounds to use for relief from tinnitus. Some of these apps also include additional relaxation and sleep techniques for managing tinnitus. Smartphone/Internet-based tinnitus treatment can be broadly divided as psychological and auditory-based treatments. The following section explains the different smartphone/Internet-based intervention programme in brief.

Tinnitus E-Programme

Tinnitus E-Programme (TEP) was initially developed for health care professionals however, it can be used with individuals with tinnitus as well. It can be used individually by the patient or with the guidance of the therapist. This programme includes tinnitus education, relaxation exercises and attentional focus exercises, mainly downloadable information and instruction sheets with digital audio files. TEP consists of six weekly modules, followed by a maintenance period of four weeks where the option to revisit the resources is open. The aim is to reduce tinnitus distress and the exact mechanism is not yet clear (Greenwell, Featherstone and Hoare 2015). The files are free to access on the website (http://www.tinnituseprogramme.org/) created for the intervention program.

Smartphone Delivered Sound Therapy

Sound therapy (i.e., masking) is a tinnitus management approach wherein, an external sound is presented to mask or cover the already present sound (Shulman and Goldstein 2010), by disturbing the attention provided to tinnitus sound and reducing the tinnitus loudness (Tyler 2006). The advancement in technology has led to the development of smartphones, through which sound therapy is easily accessible. Tinnitracks (www.tinnitracks.com) and Tinnitus Pro: Music therapy (www.promedicalaudio.com) is a tailor-made notched music therapy that claims in reducing the loudness of tinnitus. One of the major limitations of traditional non-customized masking technique, which provides a broadband noise (BBN) most classically a white noise, is that it induces masking at all the frequencies compromising for the hearing of the subject. The working principle behind sound therapy is that it suppresses the spontaneous firing happening at the level of the auditory cortex and further helps in tinnitus relief. To address these issues, Mahboubi, Ziai and Djalilian (2012) came up with a tinnitus treatment method called Harmonic Sound Therapy. It is a strategy customized specifically to provide acoustic energy which allows considerable portions of the hearing spectrum unmasked. It is also reported that a Web-based version of Harmonic Sound Therapy is effective in attaining a temporary decrease in tinnitus effects in a large number of population.

Smartphone Apps Related to Tinnitus

There are a number of apps available for tinnitus treatment in both Google's Play Store for Android devices and Apple's App Store for iOS. Kalle et al. (2018) conducted detailed research on these app stores to find those apps that claim to have tinnitus masker functionality. It was found that the major percentage of these apps had the feature of masker function in their programme. Also, other than masking features, several apps provide useful information and news of various articles, photos and videos. Other than maskers, many apps were designed to provide information to the user via news articles, videos or photos. Many apps function as more of an assessment platform, including tinnitus matching and monitoring. Very few apps included exercises aiming to treat the tinnitus via hypnosis (Kalle et al. 2018). To name a few apps, Tonal Tinnitus Therapy, Tinnitus Notched Tunes, Tinnitus Balance, Resound Tinnitus relief, Beltone Tinnitus Calmer, Tinnitus Music Therapy, Tinnitus Tuner and so on.

SOLUTIONS AND RECOMMENDATIONS

Modern technologies have great influence on the amount of collected information as well as on the quality of interaction with the patients. There are a series of studies on smartphone/Internet-based technologies as a component of clinician supervised tinnitus management as well as, self-help solutions for seekers. In both series, the major light is on awareness about the requirement of a comprehensive questionnaire that addresses contexts like tinnitus monitoring. However, there is a limited focus on the diversity of different platforms and user interfaces and the awareness about the need to cope with them. Also, as in most of the smartphone applications, the data collection and information delivery should take a platform and interface into account. There should be a connection between the assessment procedures used, the score or result obtained and with the treatment approach and level used for a more user-friendly design. It is sometimes not cost-effective for the users as it would charge more for the interaction with sensors and hearing aids. Furthermore, the user interfaces vary substantially: the design of fill-in forms, especially of those requiring free text, must be reconsidered when input is acquired through smartphones and smartwatches.

From these studies, it was found that new technologies have a great impact on the amount and quality of patient's information collected, as well as the form of interaction during this process. Many studies revolve around the smartphone and the Internet-based technologies as a part of therapist-assisted and self-help solutions for the patients. For both of these platforms, there is a requirement of awareness regarding the need for dedicated questionnaire paradigms for tinnitus monitoring and also awareness about the need to cope with the diversity of user interfaces and platforms. In line with the form of patient participation, some studies have investigated the therapist's supervision and a mix design with and without the therapist's supervision. An assessment or treatment procedure which has an option of juxtaposition would be of great deed as the patients and their problems are diverse. Hence, offering assistance when needed and providing an isolated environment as a path to self-help solutions help several patients with their therapies. The role of patient participation is naturally a central subject in these studies. There are research designs that have a high rate of attrition, thereby making the study more variable. But, with the help of new technologies, the number of patient drop-outs can be minimized with the use of eHealth/mHealth apps.

CONCLUSION

The overall goal of this chapter was to develop a framework of different smartphone- and Internet-based approaches available for both assessing and treating tinnitus. Smart technologies are gaining more popularity in the recent due to easy access to different treatment methods as well as access to remote areas. Few patients also feel more comfortable when treated in a distant mode when compared to a face-to-face approach. Studies have also indicated that there is no significant difference between the treatment using a smart technology and through traditional tinnitus treatment. Therefore, Web- or app-based technologies are considered as a good alternative in both assessment and management of tinnitus. However, there still needs to research on this aspect to know the efficacy of each of the treatment procedures on a larger population in order to comment on whether these procedures can be at par with the traditional approaches.

REFERENCES

Adams, Patricia F., Gerry E. Hendershot, and Marie A. Marano. 1999. 'Current Estimates from the National Health Interview Survey, 1996.' *Vital Health Statistics 10*: 1–203.

Andersson, Gerhard. 2015. 'Clinician-Supported Internet-Delivered Psychological Treatment of Tinnitus.' *American Journal of Audiology* 24 (3): 299–301.

Andersson, Gerhard, Pim Cuijpers, Per Carlbring, Heleen Riper, and Erik Hedman. 2014. 'Guided Internet-based vs. Face-to-face Cognitive Behavior Therapy for Psychiatric and Somatic Disorders: A Systematic Review and Meta-analysis.' *World Psychiatry* 13 (3): 288–295.

Andersson, Gerhard, and Laurence Mckenna. 2006. 'The Role of Cognition in Tinnitus.' *Acta Oto-Laryngologica* 126 (Supp. 556): 39–43. doi:10.1080/03655230600895226.

Andersson, Gerhard, Lennart Melin, Christina Hägnebo, Berit Scott, and Per Lindberg. 1995. 'A Review of Psychological Treatment Approaches for Patients Suffering from Tinnitus.' *Annals of Behavioral Medicine* 17 (4): 357–366.

Andersson, Gerhard, Tryggve Strömgren, Lars Ström, and Leif Lyttkens. 2002. 'Randomized Controlled Trial of Internet-Based Cognitive Behavior Therapy for Distress Associated with Tinnitus.' *Psychosomatic Medicine* 64 (5): 810–816.

Barnea, G., J. Attias, S. Gold, and A. Shahar. 2009. 'Tinnitus with Normal Hearing Sensitivity: Extended High-Frequency Audiometry and Auditory-Nerve Brain-Stem-Evoked Responses.' *International Journal of Audiology* 29 (1): 36–45. doi: 10.3109/00206099009081644.

Bhatt, Jay M., Harrison W. Lin, and Neil Bhattacharyya. 2016. 'Prevalence, Severity, Exposures, and Treatment Patterns of Tinnitus in the United States.' *JAMA Otolaryngology-Head & Neck Surgery* 142 (10): 959–965.

Cima, Rilana F. F., Gerhard Andersson, Caroline J. Schmidt, and James A. Henry. 2014. 'Cognitive-Behavioral Treatments for Tinnitus: A Review of the Literature.' *Journal of the American Academy of Audiology* 25 (1): 29–61.

Dallos, Peter, and David Harris. 1978. 'Properties of Auditory Nerve Responses in Absence of Outer Hair Cells.' *Journal of Neurophysiology* 41 (2): 365–383.

Davis, A., and El Refaie, A. 2000. 'Epidemiology of Tinnitus'. In *Tinnitus Handbook*, edited by R. S. Tyler, 1–23. San Diego: Singular, Thomson Learning.

Eggermont, Jos J. 1990. 'On the Pathophysiology of Tinnitus; A Review and a Peripheral Model.' *Hearing Research* 48 (1–2): 111–123.

Eysenbach, Gunther, J. A. Muir Gray, Maurizio Bonati, Subbiah Arunachalam, Thomas L. Diepgen, Piero Impicciatore, and Chiara Pandolfini. 1998. 'Towards Quality Management of Medical Information on the Internet: Evaluation, Labelling, and Filtering of Information Hallmarks for Quality of Information Quality on the Internet Assuring Quality and Relevance of Internet Information in the Real World.' *BMJ* 317 (7171): 1496–1502.

Folmer, Robert L., William Hal Martin, and Yongbing Shi. 2004. 'Tinnitus: Questions to Reveal the Cause, Answers to Provide Relief.' *Journal of Family Practice* 53 (7): 532–541.

Fortnum, H., C. O'Neill, R. Taylor, R. Lenthall, T. Nikolopoulos, G. Lightfoot, G. O'Donoghue, S. Mason, D. Baguley, and H. Jones. 2009. 'The Role of Magnetic Resonance Imaging in the Identification of Suspected Acoustic Neuroma: A Systematic Review of Clinical and Cost Effectiveness and Natural History.' *National Institute for Health Research* 13(18): iii–iv, ix–xi, 1–154.

Gander, Phillip E., Derek J. Hoare, Luke Collins, Sandra Smith, and Deborah A. Hall. 2011. 'Tinnitus Referral Pathways within the National Health Service in England: A Survey of Their Perceived Effectiveness among Audiology Staff.' *BMC Health Services Research* 11 (1): 162.

Greenwell, Kate, Debbie Featherstone, and Derek J. Hoare. 2015. 'The Application of Intervention Coding Methodology to Describe the Tinnitus E-Programme, an Internet-Delivered Self-Help Intervention for Tinnitus.' *American Journal of Audiology* 24 (3): 311–315.

Gu, Jianwen Wendy, Christopher F. Halpin, Eui-Cheol Nam, Robert A. Levine, and Jennifer R. Melcher. 2010. 'Tinnitus, Diminished Sound-Level Tolerance, and Elevated Auditory Activity in Humans with Clinically Normal Hearing Sensitivity.' *Journal of Neurophysiology* 104 (6): 3361–3370.

Hawton, Keith, Paul M. Salkovskis, Joan Kirk, and David M. Clark, eds. 1989. *Cognitive Behaviour Therapy for Psychiatric Problems: A Practical Guide*. Oxford: Oxford University Press.

Hazell, J. W. P., and S M Wood. 1981. 'Tinnitus Masking-a Significant Contribution to Tinnitus Management.' *British Journal of Audiology* 15 (4): 223–230.

Heller, Andrew J. 2003. 'Classification and Epidemiology of Tinnitus.' *Otolaryngologic Clinics of North America* 36 (2): 239–248.

Henry, James A., Christopher L. Flick, Alison Gilbert, Roger M. Ellingson, and Stephen A. Fausti. 2004. 'Comparison of Manual and Computer-Automated Procedures for Tinnitus Pitch-Matching.' *Journal of Rehabilitation Research & Development* 41 (2): 121–138.

Henry, James A., Kyle C. Dennis, and Martin A. Schechter. 2005. 'General Review of Tinnitus: Prevalence, Mechanisms, Effects, and Management.' *Journal of Speech, Language, and Hearing Research* 48 (5): 1204–1235.

Hesser, Hugo, Tore Gustafsson, Charlotte Lundén, Oskar Henrikson, Kidjan Fattahi, Erik Johnsson, Vendela Zetterqvist Westin, Per Carlbring, Elina Mäki-Torkko, and Viktor Kaldo. 2012. 'A Randomized Controlled Trial of Internet-Delivered Cognitive Behavior Therapy and Acceptance and Commitment Therapy in the Treatment of Tinnitus.' *Journal of Consulting and Clinical Psychology* 80 (4): 649.

Hesser, Hugo, Cornelia Weise, Vendela Zetterqvist Westin, and Gerhard Andersson. 2011. 'A Systematic Review and Meta-Analysis of Randomized Controlled Trials of Cognitive–Behavioral Therapy for Tinnitus Distress.' *Clinical Psychology Review* 31 (4): 545–553.

Hoare, Derek J., Victoria L. Kowalkowski, Sujin Kang, and Deborah A. Hall. 2011. 'Systematic Review and Meta-analyses of Randomized Controlled Trials Examining Tinnitus Management.' *The Laryngoscope* 121 (7): 1555–1564.

Jakes, Simon C., Richard S. Hallam, Christine Chambers, and Ronald Hinchcliffe. 1985. 'A Factor Analytical Study of Tinnitus Complaint Behaviour.' *Audiology* 24 (3): 195–206.

Jakes, Simon. C., Richard. S. Hallam, S. Rachman, and R. Hinchcliffe. 1986. 'The Effects of Reassurance, Relaxation Training and Distraction on Chronic Tinnitus Sufferers.' *Behaviour Research and Therapy* 24 (5): 497–507.

Jalessi, Maryam, Mohammad Farhadi, Alimohamad Asghari, Seyed Kamran Kamrava, Ebrahim Amintehran, Suzan Ghalehbaghi, Ashkan Heshmatzadeh Behzadi, and Seyed Behzad Pousti. 2013. 'Tinnitus: An Epidemiologic Study in Iranian Population.' *Acta Medica Iranica* 51 (12): 886–891.

Jastreboff, Pawel J. 1990. 'Phantom Auditory Perception (Tinnitus): Mechanisms of Generation and Perception.' *Neuroscience Research* 8 (4): 221–254.

Jastreboff, Pawel J. 1995. 'Tinnitus as a Phantom Perception: Theories and Clinical Implications.' In *Mechanisms of Tinnitus*, edited by J. Vernon and A. R. Moller, 73–94. Boston, MA: Allyn & Bacon.

Jastreboff, Pawel. J., J. W. P. Hazell, and J. A. Vernon. 1998. 'Treatment of Tinnitus Based on a Neurophysiological Model.' In *Tinnitus Treatment and Relief*, edited by J. Vernon, 201–217. Boston, MA: Allyn & Bacon.

Jun, Hyung Jin, and Moo Kyun Park. 2013. 'Cognitive Behavioral Therapy for Tinnitus: Evidence and Efficacy.' *Korean Journal of Audiology* 17 (3): 101.

Kalle, Sven, Winfried Schlee, Rüdiger C. Pryss, Thomas Probst, Manfred Reichert, Berthold Langguth, and Myra Spiliopoulou. 2018. 'Review of Smart Services for Tinnitus Self-Help, Diagnostics and Treatments.' *Frontiers in Neuroscience* 12: 541. doi: 10.3389/fnins.2018.00541.

Khedr, Eman M., Mohamed A. Ahmed, Ola Ahmed Shawky, Enass Sayed Mohamed, Ghada S. El Attar, and Khaled A. Mohammad. 2010. 'Epidemiological Study of Chronic Tinnitus in Assiut, Egypt.' *Neuroepidemiology* 35 (1): 45–52.

KochKin, Sergei, Richard Tyler, and Jennifer Born. 2011. 'MarkeTrak VIII: The Prevalence of Tinnitus in the United States and the Self-Reported Efficacy of Various Treatments.' *Hearing Review* 18 (12): 10–27.

Mahboubi, Hossein, Kasra Ziai, and Hamid R Djalilian. 2012. 'Customized Web-Based Sound Therapy for Tinnitus.' *International Tinnitus Journal* 17 (1): 26–30.

Marks, Isaac M., Kate Cavanagh, and Lina Gega. 2007. *Hands-on Help: Computer-aided Psychotherapy*. Hove: Psychology Press.

Martin, W. H. 1995. 'Spectral Analysis of Brain Activity in the Study of Tinnitus.' In *Mechanisms of Tinnitus*, edited by J. Vernon and A. R. Moller, 163–179. Boston, MA: Allyn & Bacon.

Martinez-Devesa, P., R. Perera, M. Theodoulou, and A. Waddell. 2010. 'Cognitive Behavioural Therapy for Tinnitus.' *The Cochrane Database System Reviews* (9): CD005233. doi: 10.1002/14651858.CD005233.pub3.

McCracken, Lance M. 1998. 'Learning to Live with the Pain: Acceptance of Pain Predicts Adjustment in Persons with Chronic Pain.' *Pain* 74 (1): 21–27.

Meikle, Mary, and E. Taylor-Walsh. 1984. 'Characteristics of Tinnitus and Related Observations in over 1800 Tinnitus Clinic Patients.' *The Journal of Laryngology & Otology* 98 (S9): 17–21.

Møller, Aage R. 2003. 'Pathophysiology of Tinnitus' 36: 249–66. doi: 10.1016/S0030–6665(02)00170–6.

Nondahl, David M., Karen J. Cruickshanks, Dayna S. Dalton, Barbara E. K. Klein, Ronald Klein, Carla R. Schubert, Ted S. Tweed, and Terry L. Wiley. 2007. 'The Impact of Tinnitus on Quality of Life in Older Adults.' *Journal of the American Academy of Audiology* 18 (3): 257–266.

Nondahl, David M., Karen J. Cruickshanks, Guan-Hua Huang, Barbara E. K. Klein, Ron Klein, F. Javier Nieto, and Ted S. Tweed. 2011. 'Tinnitus and Its Risk Factors in the Beaver Dam Offspring Study.' *International Journal of Audiology* 50 (5): 313–320.

Nondahl, David M., Karen J. Cruickshanks, Terry L. Wiley, Ronald Klein, Barbara E. K. Klein, and Ted S. Tweed. 2002. 'Prevalence and 5-Year Incidence of Tinnitus among Older Adults: The Epidemiology of Hearing Loss Study.' *Journal of the American Academy of Audiology* 13 (6): 323–331.

Ochi, Kentaro, and Jos J. Eggermont. 1996. 'Effects of Salicylate on Neural Activity in Cat Primary Auditory Cortex.' *Hearing Research* 95 (1–2): 63–76.

Park, R. J., and J. D. Moon. 2014. 'Prevalence and Risk Factors of Tinnitus: The Korean National Health and Nutrition Examination Survey 2010–2011, a Cross-sectional Study.' *Clinical Otolaryngology* 39 (2): 89–94.

Portnuff, Cory D. F. 2016. 'Reducing the Risk of Music-Induced Hearing Loss from Overuse of Portable Listening Devices: Understanding the Problems and Establishing Strategies for Improving Awareness in Adolescents.' *Adolescent Health, Medicine and Therapeutics* 7: 27.

Pryss, Rüdiger, Manfred Reichert, Jochen Herrmann, Berthold Langguth, and Winfried Schlee. 2015. 'Mobile Crowd Sensing in Clinical and Psychological Trials—a Case Study.' In 2015 IEEE 28th International Symposium on Computer-Based Medical Systems (CBMS), Sao Carlos, 22–25 June 2015, pp. 23–24. doi:10.1109/CBMS.2015.26

Pryss, Rüdiger, Manfred Reichert, Berthold Langguth, and Winfried Schlee. 2015. 'Mobile Crowd Sensing Services for Tinnitus Assessment, Therapy, and Research.' In 2015 IEEE International Conference on Mobile Services, New York, NY, 27 June–02 July 2015, pp. 352–359. doi: 10.1109/MobServ.2015.55.

Quaranta, A, G. Assennato, and V. Sallustio. 1996. 'Epidemiology of Hearing Problems among Adults in Italy.' *Scandinavian Audiology. Supplementum* 42: 9–13.

Sandlin, Robert E., and Robert J. Olsson. 1999. 'Evaluation and Selection of Maskers and Other Devices Used in the Treatment of Tinnitus and Hyperacusis.' *Trends in Amplification* 4 (1): 6–26.

Schickler, Marc, Rüdiger Pryss, Manfred Reichert, Johannes Schobel, Berthold Langguth, and Winfried Schlee. 2016. 'Using Mobile Serious Games in the Context of Chronic Disorders: A Mobile Game Concept for the Treatment of Tinnitus.' In 2016 IEEE 29th International Symposium on Computer-Based Medical Systems (CBMS), 343–348. doi: 10.1109/CBMS.2016.9

Schickler, Marc, Manfred Reichert, Rüdiger Pryss, Johannes Schobel, Winfried Schlee, and Berthold Langguth. 2015. *Entwicklung Mobiler Apps: Konzepte, Anwendungsbausteine Und Werkzeuge Im Business Und E-Health.* New York City, NY: Springer.

Schlee, Winfried, Rüdiger C Pryss, Thomas Probst, Johannes Schobel, Alexander Bachmeier, Manfred Reichert, and Berthold Langguth. 2016. 'Measuring the Moment-to-Moment Variability of Tinnitus: The TrackYourTinnitus Smart Phone App.' *Frontiers in Aging Neuroscience* 8: 294.

Shargorodsky, Josef, Gary C. Curhan, and Wildon R. Farwell. 2010. 'Prevalence and Characteristics of Tinnitus among US Adults.' *The American Journal of Medicine* 123 (8): 711–718.

Shulman, Abraham, and Barbara Goldstein. 2010. 'Principles of Tinnitology: Tinnitus Diagnosis and Treatment a Tinnitus-Targeted Therapy.' *International Tinnitus Journal* 16 (1): 73–85.

Sindhusake, Doungkamol, Paul Mitchell, Philip Newall, Maryanne Golding, Elena Rochtchina, and George Rubin. 2003. 'Prevalence and Characteristics of Tinnitus in Older Adults: The Blue Mountains Hearing Study: Prevalencia y Características Del Acúfeno En Adultos Mayores: El Estudio de Audición Blue Mountains.' *International Journal of Audiology* 42 (5): 289–294.

Stypulkowski, Paul H. 1990. 'Mechanisms of Salicylate Ototoxicity.' *Hearing Research* 46 (1–2): 113–145.

Tunkel, David E., Carol A. Bauer, Gordon H. Sun, Richard M. Rosenfeld, Sujana S. Chandrasekhar, Eugene R. Cunningham Jr, Sanford M. Archer, Brian W. Blakley, John M. Carter, and Evelyn C. Granieri. 2014. 'Clinical Practice Guideline: Tinnitus.' *Otolaryngology–Head and Neck Surgery* 151 (2_supp.): S1–40.

Tyler, Richard S. 2006. 'Neurophysiological Models, Psychological Models, and Treatments for Tinnitus.' In *Tinnitus Treatment: Clinical Protocols*, edited by Richard S. Tyler, 1–22. New York: Thieme.

Tyler, Richard S., Claudia Coelho, and William Noble. 2006. 'Tinnitus: Standard of Care, Personality Differences, Genetic Factors.' *ORL* 68 (1): 14–22.

Vowles, Kevin E., and Lance M. McCracken. 2008. 'Acceptance and Values-Based Action in Chronic Pain: A Study of Treatment Effectiveness and Process.' *Journal of Consulting and Clinical Psychology* 76 (3): 397.

Vowles, Kevin E., Lance M. McCracken, and Christopher Eccleston. 2007. 'Processes of Change in Treatment for Chronic Pain: The Contributions of Pain, Acceptance, and Catastrophizing.' *European Journal of Pain* 11 (7): 779–787.

Westin, Vendela, Steven C. Hayes, and Gerhard Andersson. 2008. 'Is It the Sound or Your Relationship to It? The Role of Acceptance in Predicting Tinnitus Impact.' *Behaviour Research and Therapy* 46 (12): 1259–1265.

Westin, Vendela Zetterqvist, Mikael Schulin, Hugo Hesser, Marianne Karlsson, Reza Zare Noe, Ulrike Olofsson, Magnus Stalby, Gisela Wisung, and Gerhard Andersson. 2011. 'Acceptance and Commitment Therapy versus Tinnitus Retraining Therapy in the Treatment of Tinnitus: A Randomised Controlled Trial.' *Behaviour Research and Therapy* 49 (11): 737–747.

Wicksell, Rikard K., Lennart Melin, Mats Lekander, and Gunnar L. Olsson. 2009. 'Evaluating the Effectiveness of Exposure and Acceptance Strategies to Improve Functioning and Quality of Life in Longstanding Pediatric Pain–a Randomized Controlled Trial.' *Pain* 141 (3): 248–257.

Wu, Vincent, Bonnie Cooke, Susan Eitutis, Matthew T. W. Simpson, and Jason A. Beyea. 2018. 'Approach to Tinnitus Management.' *Canadian Family Physician* 64 (7): 491–495.

Tele-Special Education for Communication Disorders in India

Yashaswini R. and G. Malar

INTRODUCTION

India has been one of the countries to initiate specialized educational services for children with disabilities as early as the mid-1800s in the pre-independent colonial India by enthusiastic philanthropists, missionary institutions and enterprising caregivers. The first official acknowledgement of education of children with special needs in India was the report on the third Indian Education Commission. It highlighted the need for educating children with disabilities not only on humanitarian grounds but also on the grounds of utility intending to make them useful citizens (Kothari 1966). Since then the country has seen progressive changes in the field of special education, one of which is the official introduction of the integrated education programme in 1974. Later the integrated education programme was subjected to constant refinement and evolution till 1992. These endeavours eventually metamorphosed into proactive processes promoting inclusive education since 1998 under the aegis of District Primary Education Programme which was the forerunner to the Sarva Shiksha Abhiyan. Since 2009 these efforts have been extended to the secondary level of education through the scheme for Inclusive Education of the Disabled at Secondary Stage under the Rashtriya Madhyamik Siksha Abhiyan. On paper, inclusive education is ideal for ever-growing demands against dwindling resources and the pluralistic fabric of Indian educational scenario and should be able to meet basic educational needs of the massive 50 lakhs of children with special needs in the school-going age range (Kohama 2012; Thakkar 2018).

However, ground realities are strikingly different. Some 38 per cent of these children are said to be out of school, while of remaining 62 per cent, around 95 per cent of these children with special needs were enrolled in mainstream schools at least at one point of their school life while another 5 per cent were placed in schools. That is out of the total number of children with special needs in the country that only around 59 per cent received education in mainstream schools. Several of these children were reported to physically attend schools without any functional learning taking place and eventually found to stagnate or drop out over the schools years (Human Development Unit, World Bank 2009). Such degeneration arises from underplay of myriad deficiencies in the mainstream learning environment, such as inadequate policies and ineffective inclusion, uneven distribution of facilities in urban over rural locales (Kalyanpur 2008), the indifference of teachers and peers and irrelevant curricula and execution through inappropriate instructional strategies (Hegarty and Alur 2002). However, the predominant grounds cited for the disadvantaged scenario is the lack of availability of trained special educational human resources in remote and rural locales where only 15 per cent of the services are said to be distributed while more than 75 per cent of the children in need of services are resident in these places (Kohama 2012).

In this background, teledistribution of human resources and services were considered as a viable alternative with the rapid expansion of information and communication technology (ICT) across the globe especially in fast-developing communities such as India (Smith 1978; Banerjee 2014).

By definition, telepractice is the application of telecommunication technologies for the delivery of professional speech-language pathology and audiology services at a distance by linking the clinician to the client or the clinician to the other clinician for assessment and intervention and/or consultation (ASHA 2017).

Factors such as rapid development in technology, the audio-visual nature of the interaction between the clinician and the client in availing speech-language pathology services, and equitable access make delivery of speech-language pathology services eminently suitable for telepractice (Theodoros 2013). Timely deliveries of services, fewer cancellations, service delivery in the natural environment (Cason 2011) are added advantages of telepractice.

A striking similarity between speech-language pathology services and special education services is in terms of extensive use of audio-visual modality for training the targeted skills and that a major chunk of the clientele in both professions is formed by school-going children with special needs. Considering these commonalities, the delivery of special education services can be viewed as a potential area for telepractice.

Telepractice is a swiftly emerging field globally. Upper-middle income countries like Australia, the United States of America have already started using telepractice extensively. Australia, titled as one of the international 'early adopters' of telepractice has the federal government funding for the Royal Institute for Deaf and Blind Children (RIDBC) to initiate the teleschool programme. The programme has a provision to install dedicated videoconferencing equipment in homes to facilitate interaction between practitioners and families of children who are deaf and hard of hearing (McCarthy 2011). Thus, significant time, efforts and funds are invested at the federal government level to promote telepractice in Australia. Across the United States, speech-language pathologists and audiologists seem to be adopting telepractice enthusiastically. For instance, in ASHA's Special Interest Group (SIG) 18, telepractice, grew to over 1,000 affiliates in its first four years of existence; telepractice was a discrete topic in 2015 ASHA convention (Brown, 2014).

Survey studies on telepractice carried out in the United States of America reveal interesting results. A telephonic survey was conducted to assess the use of telepractice among audiologists and speech-language pathologists (SLPs; ASHA 2002). Among the 1,667 respondents, 842 (50.5%) were audiologists and 825 (49.5%) were SLPs. One-tenth (11%) of the respondents used telepractice in which 12 per cent were audiologists and 9 per cent were SLPs. The study revealed barriers to the use of telepractice as perceived and indicated by the respondents: cost (14%), lack of professional standards (13%), lack of data on efficacy cost-effectiveness (11%), reimbursement policies (7%), concern about malpractice liability (7%), concern about patient confidentiality (6%), licensure laws that affect interstate practice (5%), other factors (76%). On further analysis of 'other factors', 22 per cent reported a need for more information about what telepractice entails, 16 per cent felt it would be detrimental to the quality of service, 14 per cent felt telepractice to be inappropriate dealing with small children or patients with disabilities that required hands-on services.

On similar lines, another Web-based survey in 2014 on behalf of SIG 18 was fielded (Brown 2014). 1,713 individuals who were either current SIG 18 affiliates and/or who had indicated 'telepractice/telehealth' as an area of expertise on the ASHA dues notice were considered. Among the respondents, 85.2 per cent were clinical service providers in speech-language pathology and only 9.5 per cent provided services in audiology. Similar to ASHA 2002 study, not all respondents were tele-practitioners. However, a greater percentage of participants used telepractice model of service delivery, including 51.9 per cent of respondents who provided audiology services and 55.4 per cent who provided speech-language pathology services. Respondents were from across the states of the United States. The results revealed that, apart from delivering services to clients in their own and neighbouring states, 38 participants indicated that they provided teleservices outside of US in which 7 provided services to India. The types of facilities in which SLPs served through telepractice included pre-elementary/elementary/secondary/residential schools, clients' homes, colleges/universities, medical hospitals, rehabilitation hospitals, SLPs' office/clinics. SLPs served individuals from all age groups and carried out assessment, treatment, follow up/monitoring, professional consultation through telepractice. These services were provided mostly to individuals with language disorders, articulation and phonological disorders, fluency disorders, autism spectrum disorder, motor speech disorders, cognitive-communicative disorders, learning disabilities, voice/resonance disorders, literacy, aphasia and many more conditions. The most frequent barrier reported by 48.4 per cent of the SLPs was licensure requirement both at home and at the place where client is located. 56 per cent of the SLPs responded that they received reimbursement for telepractice. 37.4 per cent SLPs felt that there are adequate consumer protections currently in place in their respective state for patients/clients to be properly treated via telepractice for audiology and/or speech-language pathology. This study in contrast to the study by ASHA in 2002 had more respondents who were SLPs using telepractice model of service delivery than audiologists. The study further explored reimbursement policies. The study provided evidence that more than 56 per cent of the SLPs receive reimbursement for telepractice. Although the former study revealed that Licensure laws affect interstate practice, the later study revealed that this did not prevent SLPs from delivering telepractice to other states and outside the USA. Thus, brought to the light both perspective of SLPs and audiologists and the practical scenario in terms of interstate licensure, consumer protection, reimbursement in telepractice. These studies explored and pointed out barriers to telepractice. The respondents were speech-language pathologists and audiologists, so studies exploring perspectives and perceptions on telepractice of special educators were warranted.

In an attempt to explore the perspectives on professionals delivering teleservices in a school setting, a survey was carried out considering 170 school-based SLPs (Tucker 2012a). Among the participants, only 1.8 per cent of the participants reported to used telepractice in school-settings. The core questions of the survey were designed to elicit responses on a Likert scale. The survey led to some interesting facts such as willingness to use telepractice was inversely related to age. The study revealed that telepractice model of service delivery was offered to provide screening, assessment, treatment and consultation to the children with language disorder (71.4%); articulation/phonology (1%); fluency (28.6%); learning disabilities; autism spectrum disorders, and attention deficit (14.2%). Majority of the respondents (71.4%) believed that all areas in speech-language pathology were suitable for telepractice. However, there were respondents who differed in their belief and reported that birth to three, dysphagia or motor speech disorders (57.1%); articulation/phonology, autism spectrum disorders, fluency or preschool (42.8%), hearing impairment, mental retardation, psychiatric/emotional disturbances or voice (28.6%); learning disabilities (14.2%) were the areas not suitable for telepractice. As did the respondents of the previous survey (ASHA 2002), concerns about the validity of assessments administered via telepractice; rapport building with clients via telepractice; effectiveness of telepractice in relation to in-person speech-language therapy were expressed. In addition, most respondents indicated a need to establish procedures and guidelines for school-based telepractice programs. In continuation with this study, Tucker in the same year reported the experiences, attitudes and beliefs regarding specific elements of telepractice in schools in another publication (Tucker 2012b). It was a qualitative study of the responses to a telephonic interview from five participants, experienced in tele-speech-language pathology in school settings. Unlike the studies mentioned earlier which included responses from both those delivering services through telepractice and face-to-face model of service delivery, the study considered participants using only telepractice model of speech-language pathology service delivery. The participants dealt with children from preschool to high school and served children with deficits in articulation, fluency/ stuttering, language, learning disability, pervasive developmental disorder, autism spectrum disorder, central auditory processing disorder, children who used augmentative and alternative communication. The services provided comprised of screenings, assessments, individualized education programme meetings, therapy, consultations with teachers and bilingual therapy. Technology failure in terms of interruption in network, failure/breakdown of the hardware or transducers used for telepractice was the most frequently reported barrier to telepractice, in addition, absence of technical support was pointed out as another hurdle. Inadequate training in the technical aspects to handle the equipment and procedures for telepractice was reported as a bigger challenge in telepractice than the actual specific training strategy itself. Another related hurdle was untrained E-helpers or assistants at the client's end resulting in ineffective assistance to students in terms of technical aspects or otherwise, thus deficits in training extended to these as well. The lack of specified procedures to guide smooth telepractice programming was reported as the next frequently-cited barrier. Lack of physical contact with students for implementation of the traditional articulation therapy, physical redirection such as hand over hand manipulation was reported as another barrier to telepractice besides treating children with sensory impairments, severe to profound cognitive impairments, apraxia, voice, dysphagia, severe psychological problems and children who used alternative and augmentative communication. The respondents indicated that ethics, confidentiality and privacy of telepractice in school settings were to be considered before initiating telepractice. The survey also shed light on benefits of telepractice in school settings. Access to speech-language pathology services to remote and underserved areas, individualized programming for each student was felt more effective via telepractice as students were independent to avail services. The telepractice model made the service delivery more intense and personal, gave room for specialized services in two languages when the SLPs were bilingual; greater acceptance from the students as they were motivated by the use of computer and technology (Tucker 2012b).

Taking experience from the upper-middle income countries, India is also embracing the tele-model of service delivery in the field of speech-language pathology and special education. To explore the awareness, the viability of service delivery, the requirement of certification and infrastructure required for telepractice, a survey was conducted on SLPs and audiologists in India (Mohan et al. 2017). 2800 SLPs and audiologists registered with the Indian Speech and Hearing Association (ISHA) were considered for the questionnaire survey. Totally, 205 SLPs and audiologists responded to the questionnaire. 87.80 per cent (n = 180) of the respondents provided in-person service delivery (Group II) and 12.19 per cent (n = 25) of the respondents were tele-practitioners (Group I). Among respondents in Group II, 55 per cent (n = 172) were aware of telepractice. Ninety percent (n = 162) perceived that telepractice can be a viable form of service delivery; 73.3 per cent (n = 132) opined that the professionals must be certified for telepractice; and 81.66 per cent (n = 147) stated that the infrastructure required for service delivery through telepractice is different from conventional in-person service delivery. 92 per cent (n = 166) expressed that there is an inadequate number of telepractice providers in their respective states in India. In addition, 83.90 per cent (n = 151) respondents believed that sufficient resources are not available for telepractice. Most, 92.68 per cent (n = 167) were of the opinion that legal guidelines are needed for telepractice in India. The respondents in group I also believed there is an inadequate number of telepractice providers in their respective states India (Mohan et al. 2017).

Another questionnaire survey was carried out on tele-SLPs in India (Yashaswini and Rao 2018). The survey reported technical issues as barriers to telepractice. In addition, face-to-face and telemodel of speech language pathology service delivery was reported to be different in terms of instructions for caregivers, documentation, face validity, acceptance and responsibility on caregivers. It was also reported that more sensitivity and caution, special ICT skills for clinicians and caregivers/clients, exclusive software, dedicated professionals to troubleshoot technical issues are additional requirements for telepractice. Concerns about client confidentiality were expressed and lack of direct feedback and environmental distractions at clients' end were reported as challenges in telepractice delivery. The study concluded that service delivery through telemodel is mostly positively embraced in India, despite the challenges.

Thus, research in India considering both professionals using face-to-face model and telemodel of speech-language pathology service delivery have revealed mostly positive attitudes. In addition, telepractitioners have also reported additional skills and concerns for telepractice in the field of speech-language pathology. Considering the dearth of literature in the field of special education, the present study aims to explore the perspectives, perceptions and perceived competence of educators on telepractice for delivery of special education services.

METHODS

The present study aimed to evaluate the perceptions (knowledge), perspectives (attitudes), and perceived competence in telepractice among special educators. This was in view of exploring the knowledge (12 items), attitudes (10 items) and assumed competence (10 items) of special educators to deliver special education services through telepractice. For the purpose, a survey using a questionnaire was conducted.

PARTICIPANTS

In total 50 participants between the age of 24–54 years responded to the questionnaire. All participants were from the states of Karnataka and Kerala of South India, working in both government and non-government organization. The respondents had exposure to handling children with a wide variety of communication disorders and had worked in a variety of settings including school setting, clinical setting, vocational setting and a combination of two or more. They delivered their services to children with special needs at different academic levels. The number of years of the experience of the respondents varied from less than 5 years to more than 20 years. The respondents had a minimum qualification of Diploma in Special Education to Doctoral degree in special education. The specific details of the socio-demographic details are presented in Table 8.1 and elaborated in the results section.

RESEARCH DESIGN

The present study used survey research design and used a questionnaire for the purpose. The questionnaire was emailed to the four participants with instructions along with the consent form. A printed questionnaire was distributed to 49 participants who consented to participate in the study and the filled in questionnaires were collected. The responses from the participants were kept confidential. The initial part of the questionnaire elicited socio-demographic details. The body of the questionnaire had 32 questions under three headings. 12 items under the heading of perception of educators towards telepractice elicited a response on knowledge towards telerehabilitation through binary choice questions with 'yes' and 'no' as choices. Another column named remarks elicited the reason or any comments related to the response to the test items. 10 items under the heading of perception of educators towards telerehabilitation elicited responses on the attitudes towards telepractice of the respondents. This section also had a provision for the respondents to record any comment or remarks relevant to the answer for the particular question. 10 items under the heading of perceived competence elicited a response on skills that are necessary for the delivery of special education service through telemodel of service delivery on a 3-point rating scale. The three points on the rating scale were highly competent, partially competent and incompetent.

Table 8.1 Socio-demographic Details of the Respondents

Age/Gender	Type of Organization	Exposure to Children with Special Needs	Professional Qualification	Nature of Work Setting	No. of Years of Experience	Level of Teaching
Age range—24 to 54 years (M = 34.4 years, SD—6.45).	Government (n = 16, 32%)	Communication disorders (ADHD, ASD, CP, ID, LD, HI, & multiple disabilities) (n = 15, 30%)	Diploma in early education/special education (n = 30, 60%)	School setting (n = 39, 78%)	<5 years (n = 9, 18%)	Pre-primary (n = 11, 22%)
Female n = 43 (86%)	Non-government (n = 34, 68%)	Hearing impairment (n = 34, 68%)	Graduation in special education (n = 10, 20%)	Clinical setting (n = 3, 6%)	5-10 years (n = 18, 36%)	Primary (n = 22, 44%)
Male n = 7 (14%)		Learning disability (n = 1, 2%)	Postgraduation in special education (n = 8, 16%)	Technical/vocational setting (n = 1, 2%)	10–15 years (n = 12, 24%)	Higher primary (n = 7, 14%)
			Doctoral degree in special education (n = 2, 4%)	Combination of the above (n = 7, 14%)	15-20 years (n = 6, 12%)	Secondary (n = 9, 18%)
					>20 years (n = 5, 10%)	Post secondary (n = 1, 2%)

Note: n—number of respondents, M—mean, SD—standard deviation ADHD—attention deficit hyperactivity disorder, ASD—autism spectrum disorder, ID—intellectual disability, LD—learning disability, CP—cerebral palsy, HI—hearing impairment.

PROCEDURE

The study was carried out in two stages. The first stage involved the construction of statements for the questionnaire under the heading's perceptions, perspectives and perceived competence. In addition, the initial part of the questionnaire had provision to record the demographic details such as name of the participant, age/gender, professional qualification, years of experience, level of teaching, type of organization, nature of work setting, exposure to children with special needs and contact details. Three professionals with a minimum of 15 years of experience in the field of special education/speech-language pathology carried out the content validity check. According to their reports, all questions in the questionnaire were valid. Suggestions to modify the sentence structure for two questions were given. These suggestions were considered and the questionnaire was revised. After the questionnaire was finalized in English, the same was translated to Kannada, the language spoken in Karnataka state. The final questionnaire was in bilingual format.

The second stage was data collection, the revised questionnaire was mailed to the special educators and reminders to respond to the questionnaire were sent to elicit responses from the participants. The responses from the participants were fed to IBM SPSS 20 software to run statistical analysis. Initially, descriptive statistics were run to calculate the frequency of positive attitude in percentage; frequency of correct knowledge in percentage and frequency of occurrence of perceived competence on the 3-point rating scale expressed in percentage. In addition, correlation analysis was run to explore the relationship between the demographic details and the three measures of the questionnaire.

RESULTS AND DISCUSSION

Socio-demographic Details of the Respondents

In Karnataka and Kerala states of South India, 53 special practicing educators were considered for the study through purposive sampling. Out of 53, 50 participants (94.34%) responded to the questionnaire.

The respondents were seven males and 43 females in the age ranging from 24 to 54 years (M = 34.4 years, SD- 6.45).

The respondents were experienced in teaching to students at different academic levels. Most respondents (n = 22, 44%) handled primary students, followed by pre-primary students (n = 11, 22%), secondary students (n = 9, 18%), higher primary students (n = 7, 14%) and lastly post-secondary students (n = 1, 2%).

The number of years of experience in the field of special education was categorized into five groups, 18 respondents (36%) had 5–10 years of experience, and 12 respondents (24%) had 10–15 years, 9 respondents (18%) had less than 5 years of experience, 6 respondents (12%) had 15–20 years of experience and 5 respondents (10%) had more than 20 years of experience in the field of special education.

The professional training of the respondents ranged from diploma to doctoral degree in special education. 30 respondents (60%) had a professional qualification of diploma in early childhood special education/special education, 10 respondents (20%) had graduation in special education, eight respondents (16%) were postgraduates in special education and two respondents (4%) had a doctoral degree in special education.

Out of 50 respondents, 16 (32%) were working in government organizations and remaining 34 (68%) were working in private organizations.

15 respondents (30%) had experience in handling children having a wide range of communication disorders such as attention deficit hyperactivity disorder, autism spectrum disorder, cerebral palsy, intellectual disability, learning disability, hearing impairment and children with multiple disabilities. 34 respondents (68%) had experience in handling children with hearing impairment only and one respondent (2%) had experience in handling children with learning disability only.

The nature of work setting in which the respondents had experience ranged from the school setting, clinical setting, technical or vocational setting and a combination of the above. 39 respondents (72%) had experience working in the school setting, seven respondents (14%)

had experience working in a combination of work setting, three (6%) had experience in the clinical setting and 1 (2%) had experience in a technical or vocational setting.

Perception of the Respondents towards Telepractice (Knowledge)

12 statements elicited knowledge of the respondents on telepractice. Out of twelve statements, for eleven statements, the response 'Yes' was considered as reflective of correct knowledge and for one statement, the response 'No' was considered to indicate correct knowledge. The perception in four domains were explored; firstly, knowledge on infrastructure requirements in terms of the hardware, software, Internet connection and features of the software for telepractice were examined; secondly, awareness on whether telepractice can offer provision for close observation of the response of the children with special needs, group intervention, individual attention to the children in school setting and real-time interactions with the children with special needs were examined. These parameters are essential requirements for the process of effective delivery of special education services, especially in a school setting. Knowing that telepractice can offer provisions such as above, reflects the readiness of respondents to use telemodel of special education service delivery despite the differences between face-to-face and telemodel of service delivery. The third domain evaluated knowledge on requirements from the remote end to have an adult facilitator, technically sound caregiver and exceptions for certain conditions in which telepractice is not suitable. Awareness about these aspects, places the special educator in an advantageous position because he will know the possible reasons for breakdown or failure in the service delivery, for which he will be prepared to troubleshoot or accept that some conditions are simply not suitable for the telepractice. Lastly, knowledge on whether telepractice is successfully implemented in developed nations was elicited. Compilation of responses from 50 respondents on 12 items revealed 86.17 per cent correct knowledge and 13.83 per cent wrong knowledge on telepractice. Thus, knowledge of telepractice seems to be appreciable among special educators.

Considering that knowledge is essential for practical implementation, appreciable knowledge among special educators considered in the study reflects readiness of the respondents to use telemodel for delivery of special education services in future.

Perspectives of the Respondents towards Telepractice (Attitude)

10 statements elicited the attitudes of the respondents towards telepractice. Out of 10 statements, for seven statements, the response 'Yes' was considered as reflective of a positive attitude and for three statements, the response 'No' was considered as indicative of a negative attitude. The statements mainly focused on three aspects. Firstly, whether the participants had a positive attitude about the feasibility of telemodel of service delivery in special education, specifically for mainstreamed children and incorporation of telemodel in the existing system of special education service delivery. Secondly, attitudes towards available infrastructure and skill sets for tele-special education service delivery and attitudes towards the limitation of telepractice. Compilation of responses from 50 participants on the 10 items yielded 68 per cent positive attitude and 32 per cent negative attitude towards telepractice. The results showed mostly positive attitudes among the respondents.

These results are similar to that reported by Tucker (2012a), where the majority of speech and hearing professionals (71.4%) who delivered their services in school settings opined that all areas in speech-language pathology were suitable for telepractice. In addition, major positive attitudes towards telepractice reflected in the present study are in consonance with the results reported by Mohan et al., 2017. The study reported that 90 per cent of the participants expressed that telepractice can be a viable option. The high positive attitude among special educators towards telepractice places them in a position where they can more readily deliver their services through telepractice, also convince caregivers to avail services through telepractice and promote telepractice in their work environment more easily.

Perceived Competence (Assumed Competence)

10 statements elicited a response on perceived competence on a 3-point rating scale. A score of 3, 2 and 1 were assigned to highly competent, partially competent and incompetent responses, respectively. Compilation of responses from 50 respondents on 10 items on the 3-point rating scale revealed that 54 per cent of the responses indicated high competence, 43.8 per cent indicated partial competence and 2.2 per cent indicated incompetence. Thus implying that there is scope for further enhancing the skills of special educators so that they can make constructive contributions to the education of children with special needs through teleservices.

As the incompetency for skills required to deliver telespecial education services was only 2.2 per cent, the respondents seem to be equipped mentally with the skill set necessary for the purpose. However, high perceived competence to deliver telespecial education services formed 54 per cent of response and partial competence 43.8 per cent, there is a lot of scope for the special educators to learn the skills and brace themselves to involve in telepractice.

Correlation Between Age and Number of Years of Experience of the Respondents with Perceptions, Perspectives and Perceived Competence

Correlation analysis was run to evaluate whether there is any relationship between the two variables age: the number of years of experience on the attitude, knowledge and perceived competence of the respondents. Spearman's rank-order correlation was run using IBM SPSS 20 software. The results revealed no statistically significant correlation between age and attitude of the respondents (r_s [48] = –0.105, p = 0.467); age and knowledge of the respondents (r_s [48] = 0.216, p = 0.132); age and perceived competence of the respondents (r_s [48] = –0.024, p = 0.871). Though statistically insignificant, negative correlation trend can be observed between age and attitude, age and perceived competence. Implying that, younger respondents had a more positive attitude and more perceived competence than elder ones.

The trend of negative correlation between age and attitude has been reported by several studies in the literature (Tucker 2012a; Martí-Parreño, et al. 2013, Sánchez-Mena, Martí-Parreño and Aldás-Manzano 2017). Similarly, age and perceived competence has been reported by several studies (Ahmed, Sharma and Deppeler 2014, Bornman and Donohue 2013).

Correlation analysis results revealed no statistically significant correlation between number of years of experience and attitude (r_s [48] = -0.089, p = 0.538); number of years of experience and knowledge (r_s [48] = 0.037, p = 0.801); number of years of experience and perceived competence (r_s [48] = -0.032, p = 0.825). Negative correlation trend can be noted between the number of years of experience and attitude; and between the number of years of experience and perceived competence. Implying that, a greater number of years of experience does not relate to a more positive attitude or better-perceived competence.

SUMMARY AND CONCLUSION

The country is running low on the human resources necessary for providing special education services to the children with special needs, especially in remote areas. Telepractice is one of the solutions to reach out to schools in rural areas and provide special education services to the children with special needs. However, since the concept of telepractice in India for delivery of special education services is still in an infant state. A survey was carried out to explore the perceptions, perspectives and perceived competence towards telepractice. 50 special educators practicing in Karnataka and Kerala states were considered through purposive sampling. A questionnaire with provision to record socio-demographic details and 32 statements intended to elicit the participants' knowledge, attitudes and assumed competence in telepractice were distributed to the participants and responses were compiled.

The responses on the perceptions indicated that the participants had appreciable knowledge base (86.17%) on telepractice regarding the infrastructure requirements, awareness on essential requirements for the process of effective delivery of special education services, requirements from the remote end. The participants mostly displayed positive attitudes (68%) towards telepractice. Thus, appreciable knowledge and positive attitude towards telepractice reflect the readiness of the respondents to use telemodel for delivery of special education services in future. It also indicates that these professionals are in a better position to convince caregivers to avail services through telepractice and promote telepractice in their work environment more easily.

The measure of perceived competence revealed that most participants indicated that they had high competence (54%), followed by partial competence (43.8%) and incompetence (2.2%). These scores indicate that there is scope for skills training for special educators to make them more competent in-service delivery through telepractice.

Overall better knowledge, positive attitude towards telepractice and better-perceived competence for telepractice places the special educators in an advantageous position to embrace telepractice more readily and serve more number of school-going children with special needs, thus breaking the geographical barriers and making special education services accessible to more schools. In turn, making inclusive education a practical reality.

Correlational findings demonstrate trends indicating that younger participants have a more positive attitude and perceived competence, implying more work in building positive attitudes and motivating elderly special educators to use telepractice.

ACKNOWLEDGEMENTS

The authors wish to acknowledge the permission and support received from the Director, AIISH, Mysuru. The authors are thankful to the cooperation of the Head of the Tele-center for Persons with Communication Disorders, AIISH, and participants from special schools for children with hearing impairment.

REFERENCES

Ahmed, M., U. Sharma, and J. Deppeler. 2014. 'Variables Affecting Teachers' Intentions to Include Students with Disabilities in Regular Primary Schools in Bangaladesh.' *Disability and Society* 29 (2): 317–331.

American Speech-Language-Hearing Association—ASHA. 2002. 'Survey of Telepractice Use among Audiologists and Speech–Language Pathologists.' Available at: http://www.asha.org/uploadedFiles/practice/telepractice/SurveyofTelepractice.pdf (accessed on 25 July 2017).

American Speech-Language-Hearing Association—ASHA. 2017. 'Telepractice 2017.' Available at: https://www.asha.org/Practice-Portal/Professional-Issues/Telepractice/ (accessed on 25 July 2017).

Banerjee, Gargi. 2014. 'ICT Development in India: Current Scenario.' *International Journal of Current Research* 6 (1): 4685–4689.

Bornman, J., and D. K. Donohue. 2013. 'South African Teachers' Attitudes towards Learners with Barriers to Learning.' *International Journal of Disability, Development and Education* 60 (2): 85–104.

Brown, J. 'The State of Telepractice in 2014.' *The ASHA Leader* 19 (12): 54–57. doi:10.1044/leader.FTR3.19122014.54.

Cason, J. T. 2011. 'Telerehabilitation: An Adjunct Service Delivery Model for Early Intervention Services.' *International Journal of Telerehabilitation* 3 (1): 19–30.

Hegarty, Seamus, and Mithun Alur, eds. 2002. *Education of Children with Special Needs: From Segregation to Inclusion.* Thousand Oaks, CA: SAGE Publications.

Human Development Unit, World Bank. 2009. *People with Disabilities in India: From Commitments to Outcomes.* Dhaka: South Asian Region Office, The World Bank.

Kalyanpur, Maya. 2008. 'Equality, Quality and Quantity: Challenges in Inclusive Education Policy and service Provision in India.' *International Journal of Inclusive Education* 12 (3): 243–262.

Kohama, Angela. 2012. *Inclusive Education in India: A Country in Transition.* Undergraduate Honors Thesis, Department of International Studies, University of Oregon, Oregon, 55.

Kothari, P. S. 1966. *Report of Third Indian Education Commission.* Report of Indian Education Commission, Ministry of Education, Government of India, New Delhi, 123.

Martí-Parreño, J., C. Ruiz-Mafé, Charles C. Chen, and B. Barrado-Jiménez. 2013. 'The Effect of Students' Attitude on Acceptance of and Satisfaction with a Skype-Based E-Learning System.' *Proceedings 7th International Technology, Education, and Development Conference (INTED)*, 4–6. Valencia, Spain: INTED.

McCarthy, M. 2011. 'Using technology to support children with sensory disability in remote areas: The RIDBC Teleschool model.' *Telecommunications Journal of Australia* 61: 27.1–27.7.

Mohan, H. S., A. Anjum, and Rao P. K. S. 2017. 'A Survey of Telepractice in Speech-Language Pathology and Audiology in India.' *International Journal of Telerehabilitation* 9: 69–80

Sánchez-Mena, Antonio, José Martí-Parreño, and Joaquín Aldás-Manzano. 2017. 'The Effect of Age on Teachers' Intention to Use Educational Video Games: A TAM Approach.' *The Electronic Journal of e-Learning* 15 (4): 355–366.

Smith, Delbert D. 1978. *Teleservices via Satellite: Experiments and Future Perspectives.* Alphen aan den Rijn, The Netherlands: Sijthoff & Noordhoff.

Thakkar, Amrita. 'Essential Guide to Special Needs Education in India.' *Frist Crayon.* April 27, 2018. Available at: https://blog.firstcrayon.com/the-essential-guide-to-special-needs-education-in-india–47769fc4d234 (accessed 14 October 2019).

Theodoros, D. 2013. 'Speech-language Pathology and Telerehabilitation.' In *The Telerehabilitation*, edited by S. Kumar and Cohn E. R., 311–324. London: Springer.

Tucker, J. K. 2012a. 'Perspectives of Speech-Language Pathologists on the Use of Telepractice in Schools· Quantitative Survey Results.' *International Journal of Telerehabilitation* 4: 61–72.

Tucker, J. K. 2012b. 'Perspectives of Speech-Language Pathologists on the Use of Telepractice in Schools: The Qualitative View.' *International Journal of Telerehabilitation* 4: 47–60.

Yashaswini, R., and P. K. S. Rao. 2018. 'Tele Speech-Language Pathology and Audiology in India—A Short Report'.' *Journal of International Society of Telemedicine and eHealth* 6: 1–8.

Telerehabilitation in Mental Health

2

Man with Machine or Man versus Machine? Insights from Technology-Based Rehabilitation in Persons with Aphasia

9

Vimala Jayakrishna Kasturi and
S. P. Goswami

INTRODUCTION

Information and communication technologies (ICTs) have been a driving force in overcoming barriers to access in the healthcare sector and have led to the emergence of telepractice as a means of providing cost-effective and continued healthcare. Not only does the implementation of telerehabilitation help in reducing travel time and expenses for accessing healthcare, but also benefits the patient by proving an opportunity to better adhere to the treatment programme and thereby lead to improved quality of life. However, the implementation of telerehabilitation also faces umpteen challenges (Wootton 2008). In India 20 million persons with disability have been identified out of a population of 1.3 billion. However, there are only about 3500 registered professionals in the field of audiology and speech-language

The authors express our sincere gratitude to Dr Swathi Kiran, Co-founder & Chief Scientist of healthcare start-up Constant Therapy for providing us with an opportunity to work in collaboration with their firm.

pathology in India pointing to a huge access barrier. In a survey conducted among the speech and language pathologists (SLPs) in India, it was found that only 25 SLPs were using telepractice out of a total 172 SLPs who knew telepractice could be a viable means for continued rehabilitation services (Mohan, Anjum and Rao 2017). These numbers depict the severe dearth of practitioners in India in the field of telerehabilitation. In the same survey conducted by Mohan et al. (2017), SLPs who responded to the survey were of the opinion that there is a scarcity of existing structural framework, technical support and materials to provide appropriate speech-language pathology and audiology services through telerehabilitation in India. SLPs also felt that the requirements for telerehabilitation were different from that of conventional therapy and they felt a need for formal training and certification for those who intend to implement telerehabilitation in their clinical practice. Concerns regarding the privacy security of both clinicians and clients and the availability of secured and licensed services were also expressed by those who participated in the survey. In American Speech-Language-Hearing Association's (ASHA) survey, SLPs stated that they used telehealth primarily for counselling and follow-up services and to a lesser degree for treatment and screening (ASHA 2002). Different surveys across the world attempting to identify barriers to adoption of telehealth have been carried out. One such survey by the Australian Federal Department of Health and Ageing (DHA) regarding eHealth readiness survey reported barriers to include lack of appropriate funding under medicare for allied health services, poor access to services and a lack of relevant technology (DHA 2011). In a survey on the clinical use of telehealth among SLPs in Australia revealed that the most commonly reported barriers were problems with technology (71.9%) and telecommunication connections (45.6%), closely followed by a lack of assessment and treatment resources suitable for telehealth (40.4% and 36.8% respectively).

The current study posits that software-based tele-treatment could overcome the shortcoming of lack of structured telerehabilitation programme providing the practicing clinicians with therapy material available on the app for assessment and therapy. App-based telerehabilitation like those that be implemented on a smartphone can be advantageous over other technological aids which may not be cost-effective and may not be easily available. This process of telerehabilitation permits interaction between the therapists and the persons with aphasia (PWA) through long-distance in an asynchronous manner. These help in overcoming concerns pertaining to privacy security of both the clinicians and the clients as the profile is password protected.

In the West, software programmes like CogMed, Lumosity, Sentence Shaper, Lingraphica and Sentactics are commercially available and put to use very often. The effectiveness of CogMed (Pearson Company, Scandinavia, Sweden), a software programme created for use with individuals with brain insult was tested on 18 patients with stroke for five weeks. Progress on untrained measures of working memory and attention and fewer cognitive problems were found with tele-treatment (Westerberg et al. 2007). Finn and McDonald (2011) studied 16 participants with mild cognitive impairments using Lumosity (Lumos Lab, San Francisco), an online-based tool available on the Internet, targeting attention, speed of processing, visual memory over 30 sessions. Significant training effects on working memory and visual attention were found, establishing the efficacy of the software. Though effective, software-based telerehabilitation options are limited in their functional applications and diversity of therapy tasks available.

Overcoming the limitations of restricted diversity of available therapy tasks, Constant Therapy, an iPad (Apple Inc., Cupertino, CA) software platform was developed by Kiran, Des Roches, Balachandran and Ascenso (2013). It offers an impairment-based, individualized treatment plan for persons with aphasia, who have suffered a traumatic brain injury (TBI), stroke or dementia, or children with learning disabilities or other disorders through tele-treatment. Des Roches, Balachandran, Ascenso, Tripodis and Kiran (2015) studied the effectiveness of this app-based software platform that delivers tailored therapy for PWA and found significant and positive changes in both the domains of language and cognition.

Telerehabilitation in Indian scenario is gaining popularity in the recent past. A study by Goswami, Bhutada and Jayachandran in 2012 established the efficacy of telerehabilitation of 25 sessions for a person with Broca's Aphasia using a Web camera-based system via Skype. The study reported improved participation in the treatment programme and improved language skills. Goswami and Renuka (2013) developed a Computerized Version of Manual for Adult Aphasia Therapy–Kannada (CV-MAAT-K) to remediate functional communication, repetition, comprehension and expression, naming and reading and writing. Field testing of CV-MAAT-K has established it to be an effective tool in improving the communication skills of persons with aphasia. The outcome of a collaborative project was Constant Therapy Hindi, an adaptation of the English version of Constant Therapy, for use in the Indian context (Kasturi and Goswami 2016). To make the telerehabilitation more systematic, individualized and personalized through Constant Therapy Hindi, a wide range of treatment tasks were designed based on extensive research, aiming to remediate linguistic and cognitive skills. It can be effectively used for telerehabilitation since it enables manual delivery of tasks and also allows for the user to use dynamically upgraded tasks. The programme offers an interactive interface with instructions in text, audio and video formats which can be accessed multiple times. It helps to assess the participant's performance by measuring the accuracy and latency of the responses on each of the designed tasks. The software enables the clinicians to monitor the participant's performance on each therapy task through distance mode effectively. The programme also allows for analysis and graphical visualization of the accuracy and latency of scores for every session of usage. It is available for use independently or with multiple clients, set up homework and monitor PWA progress to make better clinical decisions for a wide range of people including SLPs, academicians and researchers.

The current chapter discusses the findings of task compliance and self-directed usage of cues in an app-based rehabilitation on 18 PWA through Constant Therapy Hindi app under the purview of literacy, knowledge of smartphone usage, caregiver support and continued guidance by the therapist. This chapter attempts to answer the following questions:

1. What factors influence the therapy compliance in app-based telerehabilitation?

2. Are literacy and knowledge of usage of smartphones pre-requisites for implementation of app-based telerehabilitation in PWA?
3. Is caregiver support important in the implementation of app-based telerehabilitation for PWA?
4. Is continued guidance by an SLP essential in app-based telerehabilitation for PWA?
5. How are the cues available on an app-based telerehabilitation used by PWA?
6. Can machine-driven teletherapy work as a stand-alone therapy for PWA?

Exploring the performance of each PWA in terms of latency and accuracy on the app-based telerehabilitation is beyond the scope of this chapter and hence is being skipped.

METHOD

Ethical Approval

After obtaining approval from the institutional ethical committee and receiving informed consent, a mobile-based telerehabilitation using Constant Therapy was administered on 18 PWA. Table 9.1 lists the demographic details of the participants.

Inclusion/Exclusion Criteria

Persons with a confirmed diagnosis of aphasia after administration of Western Aphasia Battery-Hindi (WAB-H; Karanth 1980) with normal or corrected vision and hearing were recruited from three government facilities offering diagnostic or therapeutic services for PWA across three cities in India: Ajmer in Rajasthan, Mumbai in Maharashtra and Mysore in Karnataka. Pointing and tapping skills on an i-Pad were prerequisites to use the app based rehabilitation in the current study. Each of the participants was given five practice trials on a suitable task of the app to check for the presence of pointing and tapping skills. Participants who were able to point/tap on the screen of the mobile device in response to a certain question were included in the study.

Table 9.1 Details of Participants and Documented Findings

Participant	Age Group	Type of Aphasia	Post Stroke Duration	Cognitive Linguistic Profile	Aphasia Quotient	Cues Used	Tasks Compliance	Intervention Taken Earlier	Literate	Caregiver Support	SLP Guided Therapy	Uses Smart Phone
P13	A	BA	4 M	HL/LC	72.6	129%	7	No	No	No	No	No
P14	A	GA	2.6 Y	HL/HC	36	179%	9	No	No	No	No	No
P16	YA	CA	2 Y	LL/HC	41	0%	10	Yes	Yes	No	Yes	Yes
P15	OA	BA	1.5 Y	LL/HC	14.8	129%	11	No	Yes	Yes	Yes	No
P11	A	CA	10 M	LL/HC	26.6	122%	12	No	Yes	Yes	Yes	Yes
P12	YA	GA	4 M	LL/LC	0	208%	14	No	Yes	No	No	Yes
P7	A	BA	1 Y	LL/HC	9.8	195%	14	No	Yes	Yes	Yes	No
P17	A	BA	10 M	LL/HC	22.4	131%	20	No	No	Yes	Yes	No
P18	OA	BA	1 Y	LL/HC	56.6	143%	20	No	No	Yes	Yes	No
P1	A	AA	2 Y	HL/HC	57.6	123%	20	No	Yes	Yes	Yes	No
P4	OA	AA	11 Y	HL/HC	74	213%	20	No	Yes	Yes	Yes	No
P6	OA	BA	20 D	LL/HC	18	185%	20	No	Yes	Yes	Yes	No
P2	A	GA	7 Y	LL/LC	4.2	202%	20	No	Yes	Yes	Yes	No
P5	OA	GA	10 M	LL/LC	7.6	211%	20	No	Yes	No	Yes	No
P8	YA	BA	2 Y	HL/HC	54	213%	20	Yes	Yes	No	Yes	Yes
P3	A	CA	1 Y	HL/HC	53.2	199%	20	Yes	Yes	Yes	Yes	Yes
P10	YA	BA	8 M	LL/HC	20	147%	20	Yes	Yes	Yes	Yes	Yes
P9	YA	BA	1 Y	LL/LC	36	159%	20	Yes	Yes	Yes	Yes	Yes

Note: A—adult, YA—young adult, OA—older adult; D—days, M—months, Y—year; HL—high language, LL—low language, HC—high cognition, LC—low cognition; BA—Broca's aphasia, GA—global aphasia, CA—conduction aphasia, AA—anomic aphasia.

For the ease of analysis, the participants were grouped as young adults (18–40 years), adults (40–60 years) and older adults (60–90 years). The cognitive profile was assessed using informal means.

Participant Recruitment

Native speakers of Hindi who were attending speech-language therapy at the time of the current study or those who were discharged from therapy, not less than three months prior, were included in the study. The details regarding demographic data, interventions taken prior, remarks regarding family support and observations on self-motivation were recorded.

Intervention

From the domains of language and cognition, 20 tasks available on the app were shortlisted. Based on the cognitive linguistic profile of each of the PWA, a certain difficulty level of each task was assigned under each of the 20 tasks. Each PWA was required to work out five or 10 items under all of the 20 tasks selected either with the guidance of the researcher or independently after a brief period of training by one of the researchers. A total of three to five sessions, each lasting between 30 to 45 minutes were provided for the completion of the tasks by the researcher to all the participants both in face-to-face and remote conditions. Additional features of video and audio instructions aided delivery of therapy remotely.

Outcomes Measured

This chapter tries to explain aspects of task compliance and self-directed usage of cues and factors related to use or participate in telerehabilitation. The responses were recorded automatically by the app through an active Internet connection. Details like login credentials, task name, number of items attempted in each task, latency of response, the accuracy of response, number of cues used and type of cues used were recorded through the app. The task compliance was recorded by the researcher providing therapy using Constant Therapy

Hindi app. Details like years of education, whether the PWA knew how to operate a smartphone, whether the PWA has adequate family support or no and whether the therapy was delivered in person or remotely were recorded by the researcher who delivered therapy. The discussion along the lines of performance on accuracy and latency is beyond the scope of this chapter and hence are not discussed in the further sections.

RESULTS AND DISCUSSION

In an attempt to study the usage of an app-based therapy in the Indian scenario, the association between task compliance and personal factors like literacy, knowledge of smartphone usage and environmental factors like if the therapy was guided or remotely administered was explored. These measures help to evaluate if the app-based therapy programme to be effective. Task compliance is an indirect way of measuring the acceptability or usage of a certain rehabilitative measure. These inputs flag important variables to consider while implementing a therapy programme for the PWA.

TASK COMPLIANCE AND LITERACY

Among the 18 PWA who participated in the current study, 14 were literate individuals who had a minimum education of matriculation and four were illiterate with no minimal or no formal education. Out of the four individuals who were illiterate, two participants could not read or write. Of the 14 PWA who were literate, nine had task compliance of 100 per cent, and the remaining five had task compliance ranging between 75–100 per cent. Whereas, out of the four participants with minimal or no formal education, only two had task compliance of 100 per cent while the remaining two participants had task compliance of less than 50 per cent. As evident from Table 9.2, considering the total number of tasks across all PWA, the compliance was 86 per cent in the literate PWA while it was 70 per cent in the illiterate PWA.

From these results, it can be inferred that literacy was not an influencing factor in participation in app-based therapy among the

Table 9.2 *Task Compliance and Literacy*

	T1	T2	T3	T4	T5	T6	T7	T8	T9	T10	T11	T12	T13	T14	T15	T16	T17	T18	T19	T20
P8	C	C	C	C	C	C	C	C	C	C	C	C	C	C	C	C	C	C	C	C
P10	C	C	C	C	C	C	C	C	C	C	C	C	C	C	C	C	C	C	C	C
P9	C	C	C	C	C	C	C	C	C	C	C	C	C	C	C	C	C	C	C	C
P1	C	C	C	C	C	C	C	C	C	C	C	C	C	C	C	C	C	C	C	C
P2	C	C	C	C	C	C	C	C	C	C	C	C	C	C	C	C	C	C	C	C
P4	C	C	C	C	C	C	C	C	C	C	C	C	C	C	C	C	C	C	C	C
P5	C	C	C	C	C	C	C	C	C	C	C	C	C	C	C	C	C	C	C	C
P6	C	C	C	C	C	C	C	C	C	C	C	C	C	C	C	C	C	C	C	C
P3	C	C	C	C	C	C	C	C	C	C	C	C	C	C	C	C	C	C	C	C
P12	C	C	C	C	C	C	N	C	C	C	C	N	N	N	N	C	N	N	C	N
P16	N	N	N	N	N	N	N	C	C	C	N	N	C	C	C	N	C	C	C	N
P11	C	C	C	C	C	C	C	C	C	C	C	N	N	N	N	C	N	N	N	C
P7	C	C	C	C	C	C	C	C	C	C	C	N	N	N	N	C	N	N	C	N
P15	C	C	N	C	C	C	C	C	C	C	N	N	N	C	N	C	N	N	C	N
P18	C	C	C	C	C	C	C	C	C	C	C	C	C	C	C	C	C	C	C	C
P14	C	C	C	N	N	N	N	C	C	C	N	N	N	N	N	C	N	N	C	N
P13	C	N	C	C	C	C	N	N	C	N	N	C	N	N	N	N	N	N	C	N
P17	C	C	C	C	C	C	C	C	C	C	C	C	C	C	C	C	C	C	C	C

Note: Cells marked in grey indicate task compliance of illiterate PWA, cells marked in white indicate task compliance of literate PWA; C—completed, N—not completed; T1 through T20—20 shortlisted tasks for the study.

PWA who participated in this study. Contrary to the existing belief that using technology-based rehabilitation may require the person to have basic reading skills, the results from the current study demonstrated that alternative interface could replace or compliment text with audio instructions or video instructions, common symbols such that of speaker, arrow, calculator, scratchpad to work out answers as in Constant Therapy Hindi. Such supporting features in the technological aid can guide PWA towards independent usage of the app and motivate towards continuing rehabilitation.

TASK COMPLIANCE AND KNOWLEDGE OF SMART PHONE USAGE

Yet another perceived pre-requisite to participate in or use app-based telerehabilitation is the knowledge of smartphone usage. In the Indian scenario, 27.7 per cent of the total population own a smartphone (*Wikipedia* 2018). However, the details of the ownership of smartphones across various age groups is much less known. Among the PWA who participated in the current study, from Table 9.3, 11 were non-users of a smartphone while seven knew how to operate a smartphone. All the PWA in the non-users category were mostly adults (40–60 years) or older adults (60–90 years), while the users were mostly young adults (18–40 years) and a few adults. Out of the 11 PWA belonging to the non-user category, seven had task compliance of 100 per cent; two had task compliance between 75–100 per cent while two of them had less than 50 per cent task compliance. In total, there was a task compliance of 86 per cent when all sessions across the 11 PWA were considered. Among the seven PWA belonging to the user category, four had 100 per cent compliance to all the tasks; two had task compliance between 75–100 per cent while one of them had less than 50 per cent task compliance. The overall task compliance among the user group was 80 per cent.

The association between task compliance and knowledge of smartphone usage indicates that no prior knowledge of using a smartphone is required to participate in app-based telerehabilitation. Adherence to therapy was almost the same for both the users and the non-users of smartphones. One factor that may have facilitated good compliance to

Table 9.3 *Task Compliance and Knowledge of Smartphone Usage*

	T1	T2	T3	T4	T5	T6	T7	T8	T9	T10	T11	T12	T13	T14	T15	T16	T17	T18	T19	T20
P8	C	C	C	C	C	C	C	C	C	C	C	C	C	C	C	C	C	C	C	C
P10	C	C	C	C	C	C	C	C	C	C	C	C	C	C	C	C	C	C	C	C
P16	N	N	N	N	N	N	N	C	C	C	C	N	C	C	N	N	C	C	C	N
P9	C	C	C	C	C	C	C	C	C	C	C	C	C	C	C	C	C	C	C	C
P12	C	C	C	C	C	C	N	C	C	C	C	C	N	C	N	C	N	N	C	N
P3	C	C	C	C	C	C	C	C	C	C	C	C	N	C	C	C	C	C	C	C
P11	C	C	N	C	C	C	C	C	C	C	C	N	N	N	N	C	N	N	N	C
P1	C	C	C	C	C	C	C	C	C	C	C	C	C	C	C	C	C	C	C	C
P7	C	C	C	C	C	C	C	C	C	C	C	N	C	N	N	C	N	N	C	N
P2	C	C	C	N	N	N	C	C	C	C	C	C	C	C	C	C	C	C	C	C
P14	C	C	C	N	N	N	N	N	N	C	N	N	N	N	N	C	N	N	C	N
P13	C	N	C	C	C	C	N	N	N	N	N	C	N	C	N	N	N	N	C	C
P17	C	C	C	C	C	C	C	C	C	C	C	C	C	C	C	C	C	N	C	N
P15	C	C	N	C	C	C	C	C	C	C	N	N	C	N	N	C	N	N	C	N
P18	C	C	C	C	C	C	C	C	C	C	C	C	C	C	C	C	C	C	C	C
P4	C	C	C	C	C	C	C	C	C	C	C	C	C	C	C	C	C	C	C	C
P5	C	C	C	C	C	C	C	C	C	C	C	C	C	C	C	C	C	C	C	C
P6	C	C	C	C	C	C	C	C	C	C	C	C	C	C	C	C	C	C	C	C

Note: Cells marked in grey indicate task compliance of PWA who are users of smartphones; cells marked in white indicate task compliance of PWA who are non-users of smartphones; C—completed, N—Not Completed; T1 through T20—20 shortlisted tasks for the study.

therapy among non-users may have been the brief period of training by one of the researchers to teach them to use the app independently. Also, the various cues available in text, audio and video forms enable non-users to get accustomed to the operation of the app. Hence, it may be understood that, with brief exposure to new technology and cues in multiple modalities, app-based rehabilitation could be implemented across both users and non-users of technology.

TASK COMPLIANCE AND CAREGIVER SUPPORT

The researcher implementing Constant Therapy Hindi also recorded certain pertinent factors regarding the PWA participating in the study, such as if there was caregiver support while receiving rehabilitative services. These findings showed that, among the 18 PWA who participated in the study, 13 were accompanied by a caregiver who was actively involved in the rehabilitation process while five did not have any caregiver support and would attend therapy by themselves as seen in Table 9.4. When the association between task compliance and caregiver support was examined, it was found that, among the 13 PWA who were assisted by their caregivers, 10 PWA had 100 per cent compliance to therapy and three had > 75 per cent compliance to therapy. Compliance to therapy was poor in those who had no caregiver support. Among the five PWA with no caregiver support, only one had 100 per cent task compliance, one had > 75 per cent compliance while three had < 50 per cent task compliance. In terms of the total number of sessions undertaken, the task compliance was 91 per cent for the PWA with caregiver support and it was only 60 per cent for those with no caregiver support.

These findings receive support both life participation approach to aphasia as well as existing research on caregivers role in therapy specifically telerehabilitation, which posit caregiver support to be integral for rehabilitation (Palmer et al. 2013). An added finding was that younger adults and older adults were always accompanied by the caregivers, while adults were rarely accompanied by their caregivers. Restoration to work being the driving force in the younger adults, they received good support from their family and showed good task compliance. For older adults, rehabilitation served as a means of recreation than

Table 9.4 *Task Compliance and Caregiver Support*

	T1	T2	T3	T4	T5	T6	T7	T8	T9	T10	T11	T12	T13	T14	T15	T16	T17	T18	T19	T20
P8	C	C	C	C	C	C	C	C	C	C	C	C	C	C	C	C	C	C	C	C
P16	N	N	N	N	N	N	N	C	C	C	C	C	C	C	C	N	C	C	C	N
P12	C	C	C	C	C	C	N	C	C	C	C	N	N	C	N	C	N	N	C	N
P14	C	C	C	N	N	N	N	C	C	C	N	N	N	N	C	C	N	N	C	N
P13	C	N	C	C	C	C	C	N	N	N	N	C	C	N	N	N	N	N	C	N
P10	C	C	C	C	C	C	C	C	C	C	C	C	C	C	C	C	C	C	C	C
P9	C	C	C	C	C	C	C	C	C	C	C	C	C	C	C	C	C	C	C	C
P3	C	C	C	C	C	C	C	C	C	C	C	C	N	C	C	C	C	C	C	C
P1	C	C	C	C	C	C	C	C	C	C	C	C	C	C	C	C	C	C	C	C
P11	C	C	N	C	C	C	C	C	C	C	C	C	C	C	C	C	C	N	C	C
P7	C	C	C	C	C	C	C	C	C	C	C	N	N	C	N	C	N	N	C	N
P2	C	C	C	C	C	C	C	C	C	C	C	C	C	C	C	C	C	C	C	C
P17	C	C	C	C	C	C	C	C	C	C	C	C	C	C	C	C	C	C	C	C
P15	C	C	N	C	C	C	C	C	C	C	N	N	N	N	N	C	N	N	C	N
P18	C	C	C	C	C	C	C	C	C	C	C	C	C	C	C	C	C	C	C	C
P4	C	C	C	C	C	C	C	C	C	C	C	C	C	C	C	C	C	C	C	C
P5	C	C	C	C	C	C	C	C	C	C	C	C	C	C	C	C	C	C	C	C
P6	C	C	C	C	C	C	C	C	C	C	C	C	C	C	C	C	C	C	C	C

Note: Cells marked in grey indicate task compliance of PWA without caregiver support, cels marked in white indicate task compliance of PWA with caregiver support; C—completed, N—not completed; T1 through T20—20 shortlisted tasks for the study.

a rehabilitative measure. The family support continued for this age group considering their fragile health. However, the task compliance of adults was intermediate.

TASK COMPLIANCE AND SLP GUIDED THERAPY

Constant Therapy Hindi was delivered in two modes in the current study. For 15 PWA, the telerehabilitation was delivered in person through an android phone installed with Constant Therapy Hindi.

For the remaining three PWA, the installation of the app, its usage and tasks were guided remotely. The details of usage of the app, tasks performed, performance scores etc., were monitored remotely through the app itself and guidance were given over phone. When task compliance was explored among those who underwent SLP guided in-person delivered app-based therapy and remotely delivered app-based therapy, it was found that the compliance to the therapy was poor when the therapy was remotely delivered as evident from Table 9.5. There was 88 per cent compliance to therapy among those who underwent SLP guided in-person delivered therapy while it was only 50 per cent when it was remotely delivered. On evaluating other factors among PWA who underwent remotely delivered therapy it was found that two out of the three participants were illiterate, were non-users of smartphone and all three of them had no caregiver support.

SELF-DIRECTED USAGE OF CUES IN APP-BASED TELEREHABILITATION

Yet another question the current study aimed to answer was-*How are the cues available on an app-based telerehabilitation used by PWA?* To answer this, the PWA participating in the study were grouped based on their cognitive-linguistic profiles as depicted in Table 9.1. There were five PWA with High Language-High Cognition (HL-HC), nine PWA with Low Language-High Cognition (LL-HC) and four PWA with Low Language-Low Cognition (LL-LC). The usage of cues available on Constant Therapy Hindi was extracted from the app for each PWA. The percentage of cues used varies across each

Table 9.5 *Task Compliance and SLP Guided Therapy*

	T1	T2	T3	T4	T5	T6	T7	T8	T9	T10	T11	T12	T13	T14	T15	T16	T17	T18	T19	T20
P1	C	C	C	C	C	C	C	C	C	C	C	C	C	C	C	C	C	C	C	C
P2	C	C	C	C	C	C	C	C	C	C	C	C	C	C	C	C	C	C	C	C
P3	C	C	C	C	C	C	C	C	C	C	C	C	N	C	C	C	C	C	C	C
P4	C	C	C	C	C	C	C	C	C	C	C	C	C	C	C	C	C	C	C	C
P5	C	C	C	C	C	C	C	C	C	C	C	C	C	C	C	C	C	C	C	C
P6	C	C	C	C	C	C	C	C	C	C	C	C	C	C	C	C	C	C	C	C
P7	C	C	C	C	C	C	C	C	C	C	C	N	N	C	N	N	N	N	C	N
P8	C	C	C	C	C	C	C	C	C	C	C	C	C	C	C	C	C	C	C	C
P9	C	C	C	C	C	C	C	C	C	C	C	C	C	C	C	C	C	C	C	C
P10	C	C	C	C	C	C	C	C	C	C	C	C	C	C	C	C	C	C	C	C
P11	C	C	N	C	C	C	C	C	C	C	C	N	N	N	N	N	N	N	N	C
P15	C	C	N	C	C	C	C	C	C	C	N	N	N	N	N	N	N	N	C	N
P16	N	N	N	N	N	N	N	C	C	C	C	C	C	C	C	N	C	C	C	C
P17	C	C	C	C	C	C	C	C	C	C	C	C	C	C	C	C	C	C	C	C
P18	C	C	C	C	C	C	C	C	C	C	C	C	C	C	C	C	C	C	C	C
P12	C	C	C	C	C	C	N	C	C	C	C	C	N	N	N	N	N	N	C	N
P13	C	N	C	C	C	C	N	N	N	N	N	N	N	N	N	N	N	N	C	N
P14	C	C	C	N	N	N	N	C	C	C	N	N	N	N	C	C	C	N	C	N

Note: Cells marked in grey indicate task compliance of PWA without SLP guided therapy, cells marked in white indicate task compliance of PWA with SLP guided therapy; C—completed, N—not completed; T1 through T20—20 shortlisted tasks for the study.

of the cognitive-linguistic profiles. The findings suggested that the highest amount of cues were used by the LL-LC group, followed by the LL-HC group and the least amount of cues were used by the HL-HC group.

These findings provide an insight into patients' awareness of their inability to complete a language task independently (Des Roches et al. 2017). The cue usage is essentially guided by the cognitive-linguistic profile of each PWA. The groups with LL-LC and LL-HC had a lesser amount of cognitive-linguistic resources to arrive at the answers in the tasks and hence used maximal cues, whereas the HL-HC group used lesser cues.

FUTURE RESEARCH DIRECTION

Practicing SLPs must pursue research on the application of telerehabilitation to understand it better. Research along the lines of developing resources for electronic assessment and treatment and professional courses for pursuing telerehabilitation would yield significant inputs, especially in the Indian context. Human factors is an applied science that takes research about human abilities, limitations, behaviours, and processes and uses this knowledge as a basis for the design of tools, products and systems (Brennan and Barker 2008). Such findings may be helpful in designing therapeutic interventions, resource material for telerehabilitation by their professional bodies and laws and regulations for implementation by the government agencies. Though India has a national telemedicine policy, there is no mention of speech-language pathology in it. Hence, research in telerehabilitation could be pursued to lead to changes at a higher level.

CONCLUSION

The current research tried to explore factors that can affect the usage of app-based telerehabilitation and answer the following questions:

1. What factors influence the therapy compliance in app-based telerehabilitation?

2. Are literacy and knowledge of usage of smartphones pre-requisites for implementation of app-based telerehabilitation in PWA?

3. Is caregiver support important in the implementation of app-based telerehabilitation for PWA?

4. Is continued guidance by an SLP essential in app-based telerehabilitation for PWA?

5. Can machine-driven teletherapy work as a stand-alone therapy for PWA?

The results of the study revealed certain pertinent findings related to factors such as literacy, knowledge of smartphone usage, caregiver support and guided therapy which affect the participation in app-based telerehabilitation. The study posits that literacy and knowledge of usage of smartphone is not a pre-requisite to use app-based telerehabilitation provided the technological interface is user-friendly or the user has continued guidance from a caregiver or a clinician. Making the technological interface user-friendly by implementing innovative additions such as multimodal cues, facility to replay cues as many numbers of times as required, immediate feedback, graphical display of performance scores for ease of understanding helps in better compliance to the treatment thereby improving the quality of life for PWA. In consensus with earlier researches, this study emphasizes the continued support from the caregiver and positive environmental factors such as continued guidance from a rehabilitation specialist to be driving forces in participation to therapy.

To answer the final question on if telerehabilitation could be a used as stand-alone therapy, this chapter tries to emphasize that in the debate of what is effective—man or machine, one can come to a conclusion that an eclectic approach could be the best way for rehabilitation using the machine as a resource guided by an expert clinician. As evident from the findings of task compliance and caregiver support and SLP guided therapy in the current study, one can arrive at the conclusion that telerehabilitation may still require certain supporting environmental factors, essentially a sense of human touch-either by the clinician or the caregiver. The only barrier to using technology could be perceived as the technology itself. Hence, the implementation of technological innovations in telerehabilitation should be preceded by a thorough analysis and understanding of consumer experiences and needs.

Telerehabilitation can be considered an effective mode of service delivery since the primary mode of interaction is visual and verbal. Computerized programmes and apps can be an effective means to administer assessment and treatment material. However, the implementation of telerehabilitation must be based on a thorough assessment of individual needs and environmental factors and diagnosis.

APPENDIX A: CALENDAR AND LETTER TO SOUND MATCHING TASK

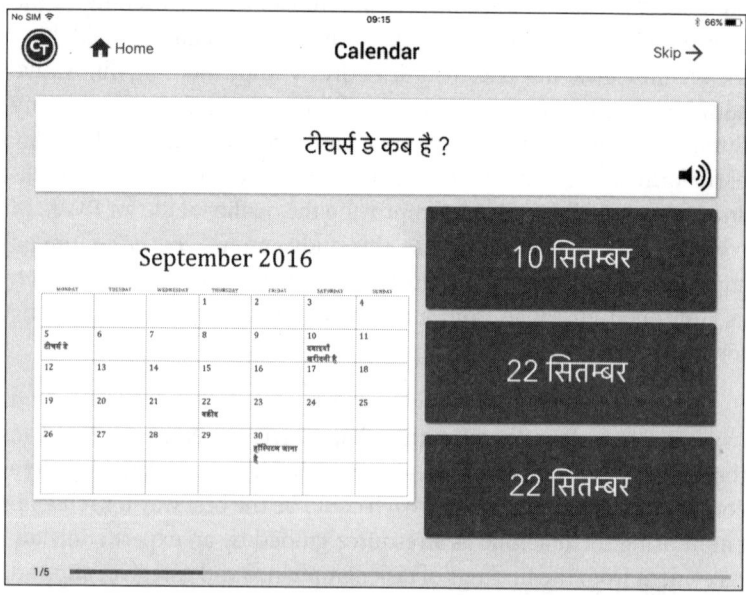

Figure 9A.1 *Calendar Task Screenshot of Calendar Task from Constant Therapy Hindi and adapted version of Constant Therapy developed by the Learning Corp. Figure obtained from version developed for field testing of Constant Therapy Hindi.*

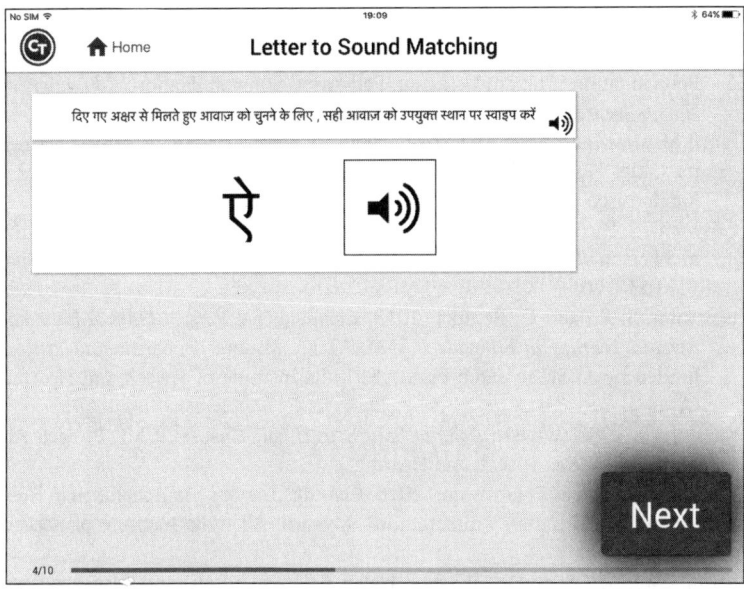

Figure 9A.2 *Screenshot of Letter to Sound Matching Task from Constant Therapy Hindi and adapted version of Constant Therapy developed by The Learning Corp. Figure obtained from version developed for field testing of Constant Therapy Hindi.*

REFERENCES

American Speech-Language-Hearing Association (ASHA). 2002. *Survey report on telepractice use among audiologists and speech-language pathologists.* Available at: http://www. asha.org/uploadedFiles/practice/telepractice/ SurveyofTelepractice.pdf (accessed on 27 December 2019).

Brennan, David M., and Linsey M. Barker. 2008. 'Human factors in the development and implementation of telerehabilitation systems.' *Journal of Telemedicine and Telecare* 14 (2): 55–58.

Department of Health and Ageing (DHA). 2011. 'The e-health readiness of Australia's allied health sector (Publications Approval Number: D0512).' Available at: https://www1.health.gov.au/internet/publications/publishing.nsf/ Content/ehealth-readiness-allied-toc/$FILE/Allied%20Health%20ehealth%20 readiness%20survey%20report.pdf (accessed on 27 December 2019).

Des Roches, Carrie A., Annette Mitko, and Swathi Kiran. 2017. 'Relationship between Self-Administered Cues and Rehabilitation Outcomes in Individuals with Aphasia: Understanding Individual Responsiveness to a Technology-based Rehabilitation Program.' *Frontiers in Human Neuroscience* 11: 7.

Des Roches, Carrie A., Isabel Balachandran, Elsa M. Ascenso, Yorghos Tripodis, and Swathi Kiran. 2015. 'Effectiveness of an Impairment-based Individualized Rehabilitation Program Using an iPad-based Software Platform.' *Frontiers in Human Neuroscience* 8: 1015.

Finn, Maurice, and Skye McDonald. 2011. 'Computerised Cognitive Training for Older Persons with Mild Cognitive Impairment: A Pilot Study Using a Randomised Controlled Trial Design.' *Brain Impairment* 12 (3): 187–199.

Goswami, S. P., Ankita Bhutada, and Kavitha Jayachandran. 2012. 'Telepractice in a Person with Aphasia.' *Journal of the All India Institute of Speech & Hearing* 31, 163–170.

Goswami, S. P., and C. Renuka. 2013. *Computerized Version-Manual for Adult Aphasia Therapy in Kannada (CV-MAAT-K).* Mysore: Departmental Project funded by AIISH research Fund, All India Institute of Speech and Hearing (AIISH).

Karanth, P. 1980. *Western Aphasia Battery in Hindi.* Mysore: ICMR Project, All India Institute of Speech and Hearing.

Kasturi, V. J., and S. P. Goswami. 2016. *Constant Therapy: An Adaptation in Hind* (Unpublished master's dissertation). Mysuru: All India Institute of Speech and Hearing.

Kiran, Swathi, Carrie Des Roches, Isabel Balanchandran, and Elsa Ascenso. 2013. 'Validation of an iPad-based Therapy for Language and Cognitive Rehabilitation in Individuals with Brain Damage.' Clinical aphasiology paper presented at 43rd Clinical Aphasiology Conference, Tucson, AZ, 28 May–2 June.

Mohan, Haritha S., Ayesha Anjum, and Prema K. S. Rao. 2017. 'A Survey of Telepractice in Speech-Language Pathology and Audiology in India.' *International Journal of Telerehabilitation* 9 (2): 69.

Palmer, Rebecca, Gail Paterson, Audrey Delaney, Helen Hughes, and Pam Enderby. 2013. 'Abstract NS14: Independent Speech and Language Practice with Aphasia Computer Software is an Acceptable Alternative to Face to Face Therapy in the Long Term Post Stroke.' In *Stroke* 44 (suppl_1). 530 Walnut St, Philadelphia, PA 19106-3621 USA: Lippincott Williams & Wilkins.

Wikipedia. 2018. List of countries by smartphone penetration. Available at: https://en.wikipedia.org/wiki/List_of_countries_by_smartphone_penetration (accessed on 17 March 2019).

Westerberg, Helena, H. Jacobaeus, Tatja Hirvikoski, Peder Clevberger, M-L. Östensson, Aniko Bartfai, and Torkel Klingberg. 2007. 'Computerized Working Memory Training After Stroke—A Pilot Study.' *Brain Injury* 21 (1): 21–29.

Wootton, Richard. 2008. 'Telemedicine Support for the Developing World.' *Journal of Telemedicine and Telecare* 14 (3): 109–114.

Telecounselling for Caregivers of Persons with Dementia

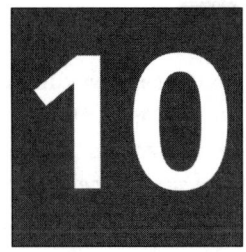

Rachel C. Francis and
Sanjeev Kumar Gupta

INTRODUCTION

In 2010, an estimate of 35.6 million people worldwide were identified as living with dementia, and by 2050, it is expected to increase three-fold (WHO 2012). According to Ferri and Jacob (2017), the greater part of the dementia population lives in low- and middle-income countries. The demographic distribution in India is changing, and the ageing population is considerably increasing. This, in turn, is going to increase the burden due to dementia in the country. According to the data on the projected increase in population with dementia around the world from 1990 to 2020, India is estimated to increase from 1.8 million to 3.7 million. According to the *World Alzheimer's Report* (Alzheimer's Disease International 2015), around 4.4 million people have dementia in India and it is expected to increase to over 10 million by 2040. Prevalence studies show that the population of dementia in lower-middle income countries is significantly higher than in upper-middle income countries and high-income countries, respectively (Alzheimer's disease International 2015). The reasons for this increase are attributed to a lack of education, which, in turn, affects cognition; culture, where women are monopolized to do certain work within the household, leading to a lack of exposure and knowledge to the outside world, which, in turn, affects cognition; lack of proper nutrition; poor diet; and increase in systemic illness (Chandra et al. 1998), not to forget the poor economic conditions making it difficult to attain quality health care services (Das, Pal and Ghosal 2012). In many parts of the country, dementia is not recognized as an illness, but rather as a part of ageing, and hence professional help is sought at a later stage of disease progression (Das, Pal and Ghosal 2012). Lack of knowledge about dementia and the stigma associated with the diagnosis delay the family seeking professional help. Health care providers are not equipped with appropriate screening tools, nor are they aware of the disease to identify it at an early stage. In most cases, caregivers (CGs) of the elderly or persons with dementia (PWDs) are spouse, non-family members or friends, while the immediate family members (children) live away from the family or abroad. Therefore, the lack of immediate familial support causes a state of emotional stress in the CGs who are spouse. In such situations, most of the parents do not express their emotions to their children. This alleviates the CG's strain, depression and anxiety. The economic burden is seen in cases where there is a lack of services available, in addition to poor economic conditions (Das, Pal and Ghosal 2012). In cases where there is a lack of monetary support from immediate family members, CGs of PWDs (CGs-PWDs) are at a disadvantage not being able to fend for themselves and PWDs. Therefore, the psychological state of CGs-PWDs calls for attention, which is mostly overlooked by the professionals involved or more so by the persons themselves. Therefore, when a person has dementia, it is not just the PWD but also the whole family that suffers (Brodaty and Donkin 2009). But the attention is seldom focussed on the CGs-PWDs. The CGs also suffer from a lack of knowledge about the condition and its care, and, in turn, undergo psychological distress.

The psychological distress present in CGs is mostly associated with the presence of behavioural and psychological symptoms of dementia (BSPDs; Cerejeira, Lagarto and Mukaetova-Ladinska 2012). The more the presence and severity of BSPDs, the higher the chances of psychological distress in CGs. The most common BSPDs in PWDs are apathy, agitation and irritability. A Chinese study (Wang et al. 2015) compared the CG distress in low- and high-income countries; it was found that the psychological distress in CGs-PWDs was higher in lower-income countries. It was also directly related to the presence of BSPDs in

PWDs. Emmatty, Bhatti and Mukalel (2006) conducted a survey to identify CGs-PWDs burden in India. They found that 30 per cent of CGs-PWDs fell into high-burden group.

CG counselling is one way of providing therapy for psychological distress in CGs. CGs-PWDs can benefit from counselling, psychotherapy and education about dementia. However, the situation is such that CGs either do not have time away from caring for PWDs or are apprehensive about leaving PWDs under someone else's care in order to attend counselling or any kind of support groups. These practical situations cause difficulty for CGs-PWDs to attend face-to-face sessions; therefore, telecounselling plays a major role in this situation. The use of technology for the assessment and treatment of the individuals is termed as telepractice. Telepractice is a mode of service delivery; it is also known as telerehabilitation, teletherapy or telespeech therapy. With the advent of technology in all the fields, the field of rehabilitation has also seen a rise in the use of apps, software and telephone intervention across various disorders. American Speech-Language-Hearing Association (ASHA) defines telepractice as 'the application of telecommunications technology to deliver professional services at a distance by linking clinician to client, or clinician to clinician for assessment, intervention, and/or consultation' (ASHA 2005). In telepractice mobile devices (e.g., iPads and smartphones), desktop computers, videoconferencing equipment and software are used. The purpose of telepractice is to make services available and accessible for all and to reach the unreached.

Telecounselling is a part of telepractice and can be email-based or text-based chat, telephone based or videoconferencing (Sussman 1998). A systematic review conducted by Scott et al. (2016) found that computer-based therapy for psychological distress in CGs-PWDs is a viable alternative for face-to-face therapy in terms of time of commute, distance to the therapy centre, availability of the professional and cost involved.

According to the Indian Speech and Hearing Association (ISHA n.d.), there are 3,347 registered audiologists and speech-language pathologists (SLPs) in the country. A global collaborative study conducted in 2016, which surveyed 195 countries, found that India alone had around 11.5 million children with developmental disability. The disability data is provided based on developmental disability alone and has not considered the acquired conditions such as aphasia, traumatic brain injury etc. Therefore, one can see the dearth of professionals available to cater to the needs of the entire disability population in the country. There is a need for more number of health care professionals to remediate the situation. One of the viable options available at hand is to make the best use of telepractice.

The beginning of telepractice in India can be dated back to exactly 10 years in 2009 by a premier central institute in South India (Rao and Yashaswini 2018). Ever since, intensive work has been going on in the areas of building awareness among and training professionals in telepractice; providing services by reaching the unreached in remote areas; and conducting audiological and speech and language assessment and rehabilitation services. The first individual to receive speech and language therapy through telepractice was a person with aphasia in 2012 (Yashwini and Rao 2018). A survey of telepractice in SLPs in 2017 found that only 12.79 per cent of respondents were involved in telepractice. Most of them used it for assessment and treatment of childhood and adult speech and language disorders but not for counselling (Mohan, Anjum and Rao 2017).

AIMS AND OBJECTIVES

Aims

The aims of the study were to find out if health care professionals are aware of psychological distress in CGs-PWDs and if they use telecounselling as a mode of intervention towards it.

Objectives

- To understand health care professionals' knowledge and attitudes towards telecounselling for CGs-PWDs
- To identify barriers in telecounselling of CGs-PWDs

METHOD

Preparation of Questionnaire

A questionnaire titled 'Knowledge and Attitude of Professionals towards Tele-counseling for Caregivers of Persons with Dementia' was created using Google Forms. The questionnaire consisted of two sections: the first included demographic details and work profile and the second consisted of questions related to telecounselling for professionals working in the area of dementia and related disorders. The second section consisted of approximately 48 close-ended questions, which were presented under subsections of attitudes, knowledge about dementia and telecounselling and barriers towards telecounselling. The questionnaire thus prepared was validated by five professionals in the area, and the inputs provided were incorporated in the questionnaire. The questions that had 95 per cent agreement were retained for the study. The final questionnaire consisted of a total of 39 questions. An outline of the questionnaire is presented in Appendix A.

Participants' Inclusionary Criteria

The participants were health care professionals within the age range of 18–58 years. In order to enhance qualitative responses, they were restricted to psychologists involved in counselling, SLPs working with PWDs and students and professions involved in telepractice. All India Institute of Speech and Hearing Ethical Guidelines for Bio-Behavioral Research 2.1e and 2.4c were followed for the current study (Basavaraj 2009). The questionnaire was circulated to 50 health care professionals via emails consisting of objectives of the survey, consent letter for participation and a link to fill in the survey. In order to preserve the privacy of the participants, the identifying information of the respondents was not collected.

Analyses of Response

The responses obtained were subjected to quantitative and qualitative analyses. The percentage was calculated for each close-ended question.

RESULTS AND DISCUSSION

Demographic Data and Use of Telecounselling

The questionnaire was distributed to 50 health care professionals, and 34 complete responses were obtained. Eighty per cent of the respondents were female. The majority of responses received were from SLPs (60%), 30 per cent consisted of psychologists and the rest were counsellors (Figure 10.1). Among these respondents, 87% of them were postgraduate, and the remaining respondents were doctoral students and professionals. Sixty per cent of them responded to have used telecounselling in their practice. On questions related to the frequency of telecounselling in the practice, only 10 per cent of them reported of using telepractice for the purpose of counselling on a weekly basis, 40 per cent used it on monthly basis and another 40 per cent never used it for telecounselling. Regarding the mode or tool used for telecounselling, majority of the health care professionals (45.5%) used emails for telecounselling, 36.5 per cent used voice over the Internet and 41 per cent used videoconferencing method; these methods have usually been the trend in telepractice. In addition, with the boom in social networking, professionals also reported the use of social media for telecounselling.

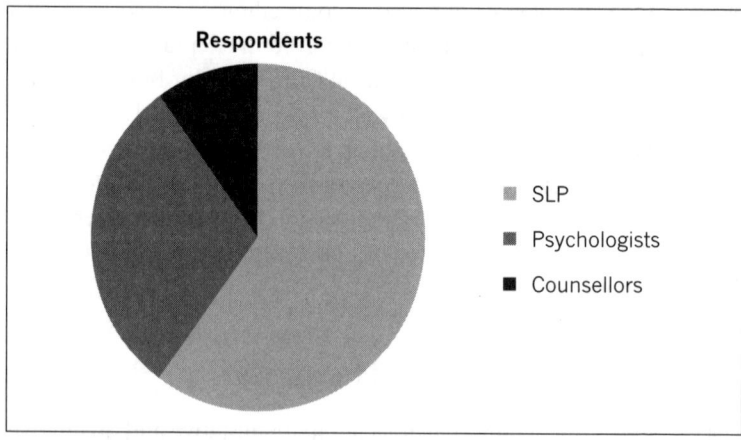

Figure 10.1 *Percentage of Professionals Who Responded to the Questionnaire*

Knowledge and Awareness of Dementia and Telecounselling

The first part of the second section of the questionnaire involved questions aimed at identifying knowledge about dementia and telecounselling among the health care professionals. Only 41.9 per cent of the total respondents reported that they were confident in assessing PWDs; the others indicated that they referred their dementia patients to their fellow professionals. Only 38.2 per cent of the professionals were aware of other telepractitioners around them, and around 26.5 per cent responded that they were not sure. Around 67.6 per cent of professionals believed that telepractice benefits patients reasoning that it reduced time and money spent on transport (82.4%). The second major reason for telepractice being beneficial was that they believed that it improved patients' continuity for therapy (67.6%). Results on close-ended questions with yes/no/maybe options related to knowledge about dementia and CGs are presented in Table 10.1. Approximately 66 per cent of them responded accurately, and 15 per cent of them were unsure about the condition.

Based on the results of this section, it can be derived that health care professionals have average knowledge and awareness of dementia. For professionals to be able to cater to the needs of CGs-PWDs to the fullest potential, there is much work to be done in the area of increasing knowledge about the condition. There is much need to increase awareness and training in telepractice so that professionals can increase the frequency of use of this mode of service delivery and with much confidence.

Barriers towards Telecounselling

The major barrier to telecounselling as reported is related to connectivity issues. The respondents also reported poor Internet connectivity to be a major barrier to using telepractice. Of the total professionals, 64.7 per cent reported that telecounselling instructions varied from face-to-face counselling, and that the patients preferred face-to-face counselling to telecounselling. Also, 82.4 per cent responded that there was a need for caution and sensitivity for telecounselling as

Table 10.1 *Knowledge and Awareness of Dementia and Telecounselling*

S. No.	Item	Yes	No	Maybe	Answer
1.	Persons with dementia are prone to depression.	76.5	20.6	2.9	Yes
2.	Persons with dementia remember recent events better than past events.	20.6	64.7	14.7	No
3.	Caregivers of persons with dementia are susceptible for anxiety and depression.	85.3	5.9	8.8	Yes
4.	Persons with dementia can benefit from psychotherapy for depression and anxiety.	64.7	32.4	2.9	Yes
5.	As the disease progresses, persons with dementia can manage activities of daily living with minimal assistance.	11.8	88.2	—	No
6.	There are adequate facilities and services available for persons with dementia in the country.	8.8	70.6	20.6	No
7.	The cost of care for persons with dementia decreases as the disease progresses.	20.6	70.6	8.8	No
8.	People in rural areas are less susceptible to dementia than people in urban areas.	29.4	38.2	32.4	No
9.	Poor nutrition can lead to dementia.	38.2	20.6	41.2	Yes

compared to face-to-face counselling. Among the other barriers for telecounselling was a requirement of knowledge about information and communications technology (ICT) and the availability of dedicated tools and software for telecounselling. A need for a dedicated technician for troubleshooting and updating the technological options for telepractice was reported by 61.8 per cent. Above all, 100 per cent of them responded that the CGs at the client end required computer knowledge to avail telemodel of service delivery. The reasons concerning barriers in telecounselling are on par with the barriers identified for telepractice in India by Yashaswini and Rao (2018). However, though people are accepting telepractice, professionals preferred face-to-face counselling to telecounselling for reasons related to privacy and lack of ethical guidelines concerning telecounselling practice in the country.

The main aim of telepractice is to reach the unreached, and it is more thoughtful towards the aid of persons in rural cities. But the digital literacy rate among rural citizens is limited, and this poses a major barrier in providing telecounselling services to the remote areas of the country. Although India has one of the world's largest growing economies, 90 per cent of the population lags behind in digital literacy (Digital Empowerment Foundation 2018). Therefore, though telecounselling sounds like an apt option for receiving counselling services in the country, it has a long way to go before it is made completely safe and achievable, acceptable and reachable to every corner of the country.

The Attitude of Professionals towards Telecounselling

Respondents rated their overall computer-related knowledge and abilities on a 5-point Likert scale, where 1 meant that they had very little knowledge and 5 meant that they had more knowledge. On average, everyone responded to have average-to-more knowledge. Only 61.8 per cent of professionals agreed that telecounselling can be effective in the treatment of psychological disorders; 23.6 per cent of them disagreed to this notion; and the rest of them neither agreed nor disagreed. Table 10.2 presents data on responses for the domain of attitude towards telecounselling among health care professionals.

Of the total professionals, 84.8 per cent believed that telecounselling would be beneficial for CGs-PWDs and PWDs. Among the professionals surveyed, less than 50 per cent (45.5%) responded to have adequate training and experiences to conduct telepractice. Forty-seven per cent of them agreed that they would use telecounselling if they had adequate training, and around 12.5 per cent responded that they would not resort to telepractice even with training, as they did not believe in the idea of telepractice. A majority of 87.5 per cent of them indicated that they were willing to attend workshops and seminars to enhance their knowledge about telepractice.

Swinton, Robinson and Bischoff (2009) found that psychologists and mental health professionals found treatment for depression through electronic mode more useful, and the patients declared that they were comfortable using more of electronic therapy. When it

Table 10.2 *The Attitude of Professionals towards Telecounselling for CGs-PWDs*

S. No.	Item	Agree	Somewhat Agree	Neither Agree Nor Disagree	Somewhat Disagree	Disagree
1.	I believe that telecounselling can be effective in the treatment of psychological disorders.	26.5	35.3	14.7	11.8	11.8
2.	I believe that telecounselling can be as effective as face-to-face therapy.	17.6	32.4	14.7	20.6	14.7
3.	I believe that telecounselling can be an effective treatment tool for some disorders, but not others.	35.3	41.2	11.8	2.9	8.8
4.	I believe that stand-alone telecounselling can be effective in providing a significant reduction in overall symptoms.	2.9	20.6	32.4	23.5	20.6
5.	If given the opportunity, I would use standalone telecounselling as an addendum to face-to-face therapy.	18.2	45.5	15.2	12.1	9.1
6.	If given the opportunity, I would use telecounselling as an addendum to face-to-face therapy.	25	50	6.3	12.5	6.3
7.	I believe that telecounselling would be better for those who have previously attended face-to-face therapy.	41.2	32.4	14.7	5.9	5.9

comes to psychological distress, people are more apprehensive about being judged when it comes to face-to-face therapy and might refrain from seeing a health care professional (Childress 2000). Therefore, obtaining information and care through electronic mode of emails, texts and voice over the Internet helps them find solace and adherence to telecounselling. This suggests that there is a need to conduct more training programmes and workshops to broaden the perspective of health care professionals to utilize telepractice more often and to be open to the idea of the same as studies have found patient satisfaction with technology-based services.

Overall, the results of the present study indicate that there are health care practitioners who are willing to expand their purview of service production by making best use of telepractice, provided they have better understanding and policies regarding the best practice method. Telecounselling is a part of telepractice. Though the majority of the professionals responded that they prefer face-to-face counselling better than telecounselling, by increasing awareness of the benefits of telecounselling, we hope to see a steady increase in the use of telecounselling.

The limitation of the study is that the majority of the responses obtained were from non-telepractice users. If the targeted telepractitioners responded, more specific information could have been obtained about the barriers and facilitators to use of telepractice for counselling.

FUTURE RESEARCH DIRECTIONS

This study only adds to the preliminary work in the country in the field of caring for the CGs-PWDs. Further research is needed to identify the type to psychological distress experienced by CGs-PWDs in India and its impact on their physical, emotional and social facets of life. Also, it would be ideal to study the kind of psychological distress experienced with different types and severity of dementia. CG expectation from counselling and rehabilitation sessions is another area that needs to be researched. The number of PWDs is increasing day by day, so the work in the area has to increase at par in order to cater to the needs of PWDs and their CGs.

CONCLUSION

Psychological distress among CGs-PWDs has been brought to the attention of health care professionals since more than a decade. In India, dementia care and awareness are in the infancy stage of development compared to other neurological conditions; thus, the CG attention is long from being tended to. Unlike most of the Western countries, PWDs in India are cared for at their homes and not in a nursing home. According to the Indian culture, sons take care of parents, and it is also considered a feminine duty to take care of the people in the house. Therefore, the primary CG is the daughter-in-law (Shaji et al. 2003). Hence, most of the CGs are obligated to provide care for the elderly as a matter of necessity and societal prejudices. The psychological distress they undergo is not considered as a primary concern to pay attention to. Moreover, CGs themselves do not realize that they need help with the anxiety and depression they are experiencing in the process of providing care to the PWDs. Therefore, caregiving stays a hidden problem with serious physical and emotional health consequences.

We, as professionals, have a long way to go in the field of dementia, starting from creating awareness among the general public, families, and CGs-PWDs and health care professionals to identifying the need and providing appropriate rehabilitation and care to the stakeholders. It is also important to take advantage of the growing digital literacy in the country to reach the rural and remote places of the country where there is a dearth of availability of direct professional contact for stakeholders. Also, it is important for institutions and organizations which are responsible for educating professionals in the area of telehealth to conduct more workshops and certificate programmes to enable confident health care professionals to take up telepractice as an addendum into their regular practice. The matters that need to be considered by policymakers in India are the privacy policy for telepractice and providing certification of telepractice to avoid malpractice or misuse of information and service delivery. It is important to know that dementia care is not equivalent to normal ageing care and needs special attention, and telecounselling presents as a promising mode of service delivery to reach the maximum number of stakeholders at ease.

APPENDIX A. KNOWLEDGE AND ATTITUDE OF PROFESSIONALS TOWARDS TELECOUNSELLING FOR CGS-PWDS

S. No.	Knowledge	Yes	No	Maybe
1.	Persons with dementia are prone to depression.			
2.	Persons with dementia remember recent events better than past events.			
3.	Caregivers of persons with dementia are susceptible to anxiety and depression.			
4.	Persons with dementia can benefit from psychotherapy for depression and anxiety.			
5.	As the disease progresses, persons with dementia can manage activities of daily living with minimal assistance.			
6.	There are adequate facilities and services available for persons with dementia in the country.			
7.	The cost of care for persons with dementia decreases as the disease progresses.			
8.	People in rural areas are less susceptible to dementia than people in urban areas.			
9.	Poor nutrition can lead to dementia.			
10.	On average, how many referrals do you receive for dementia and related disorders per month?			
11.	Please indicate the speech and language disorders you are comfortable evaluating and treating.			
12.	How many years of experience do you have as a practising professional?			
13.	Is there currently a professional using telepractice in your area?			
14.	Are you a telepractice provider?			

S. No.	Knowledge	Yes	No	Maybe
15.	Do you believe that having a telepractice provider would benefit patients that you refer to other clinicians?			
16.	What are some advantages of having a telepractice provider for dementia and related disorders in your area? (Please check all that apply.)			
17.	What are some disadvantages of having a telepractice provider for dementia and related disorders in your area? (Please check all that apply.)			
18.	Would you be interested in engaging other clinicians in telepractice if you are currently a telepractice provider?			

S. No.	Barriers	Yes	No
1.	Are there any issues in establishing Internet connectivity?		
2.	Do you think there is a difference in the usage of descriptive instructions for counselling in telemodel and face-to-face model of service delivery?		
3.	Acceptance of telecounselling by clients is similar to face-to-face model?		
4.	Does it require more sensitivity and caution in telecounselling than in face-to-face model?		
5.	Are special information and communications technology (ICT) skills required for teleservice delivery?		
6.	Is the telemodel of service delivery dependent on exclusive tools and software?		
7.	Is there a requirement of a dedicated professional to fix technical issues, and troubleshoot and update technological options available in telemodel of service delivery?		
8.	Are the caregivers at the client end required to have computer knowledge to avail telemodel of service delivery?		

S. No.	Attitudes	Yes	No
1.	I believe that telecounselling can be effective in the treatment of psychological disorders.		
2.	I believe that telecounselling can be as effective as face-to-face therapy.		
3.	I believe that telecounselling can be an effective treatment tool for some disorders, but not others.		
4.	I believe that standalone telecounselling can be effective in providing a significant reduction in overall symptoms.		
5.	If given the opportunity, I would use standalone telecounselling as an addendum to face-to-face therapy.		
6.	If given the opportunity, I would use telecounselling as an addendum to face-to-face therapy.		
7.	I believe that telecounseling would be better for those who have previously attended face-to-face counselling therapy.		
8.	I believe that telecounselling can be effective for the following: Please choose all that apply		
9.	I feel I have adequate training and experiences to conduct telecounselling.		
10.	Would you be more prone to use telepractice if you had additional/adequate training?		
11.	I believe that there is too little research on efficacious evidence-based telepractice for me to utilize such modalities.		
12.	I would be willing to attend continuing education or seminars to educate myself on telepractice.		
13.	If you do not endorse telecounselling, which is the primary concern? Please choose all that apply.		

REFERENCES

Alzheimer's Disease International. 2015. *World Alzheimer Report 2015: The Global Impact of Dementia*. London: Alzheimer's Disease International.

ASHA (American Speech-Language-Hearing Association). 2005. *Speech-Language Pathologists Providing Clinical Services via Telepractice: Technical Report*.

Available at: https://www.asha.org/policy/TR2005-00152/ (accessed on 17 December 2019).

Basavaraj, Vijayalakshmi. 2009. *Ethical Guidelines for Bio-Behavioral Research*. Mysore: All India Institute of Speech and Hearing.

Brodaty, Henry, and Marika Donkin. 2009. 'Family Caregivers of People with Dementia.' *Dialogues in Clinical Neuroscience* 11(2): 217.

Cerejeira, Joaquim, Luísa Lagarto, and Elizabeta Mukaetova-Ladinska. 2012. 'Behavioral and Psychological Symptoms of Dementia.' *Frontiers in Neurology* 3 (3): 73.

Chandra, Vijay, Steven T. DeKosky, Rajesh Pandav, Janet Johnston, Steven H. Belle, Graham Ratcliff, and Mary Ganguli. 1998. 'Neurologic Factors Associated with Cognitive Impairment in a Rural Elderly Population in India: The Indo-US Cross-National Dementia Epidemiology Study.' *Journal of Geriatric Psychiatry and Neurology* 11 (1): 11–17.

Childress, Craig A. 2000. 'Ethical Issues in Providing Online Psychotherapeutic Interventions.' *Journal of Medical Internet Research* 2 (1): e5.

Das, Shyamal K., Sandip Pal, and Malay K. Ghosal. 2012. 'Dementia: Indian Scenario.' *Neurology India* 60 (6): 618.

Digital Empowerment Foundation. 2018. 'A Look at India's Deep Digital Literacy Divide and Why It Needs To Be Bridged.' *Financial Express*, 24 September. Available at: https://www.financialexpress.com/education–2/a-look-at-indias-deep-digital-literacy-divide-and-why-it-needs-to-be-bridged/1323822/ (accessed on 17 December 2019).

Emmatty, Leena Mary, Ranbir S. Bhatti, and Mathew T. Mukalel. 2006. 'The Experience of Burden in India: A Study of Dementia Caregivers.' *Dementia* 5 (2): 223–232.

Ferri, Cleusa Pinheiro, and K. S. Jacob. 2017. 'Dementia in Low-Income and Middle-Income Countries: Different Realities Mandate Tailored Solutions.' *PLoS Medicine* 14 (3): e1002271.

ISHA (Indian Speech and Hearing Association). n.d. Life membership Details as on 24.10.2019. Available at: https://www.ishaindia.org.in/life_member/24-10-2019.pdf (accessed on 17 December 2019).

Mohan, Haritha S., Ayesha Anjum, and Prema K. S. Rao. 2017. 'A Survey of Telepractice in Speech-Language Pathology and Audiology in India.' *International Journal of Telerehabilitation* 9 (2): 69.

Rao, Prema K. S., and R. Yashaswini. 2018. 'Telepractice in Speech-Language Pathology and Audiology: Prospects and Challenges.' *Journal of Indian Speech Language & Hearing Association* 32 (2): 67.

Scott, Jennifer L., Sarah Dawkins, Michael G. Quinn, Kristy Sanderson, Kate-Ellen J. Elliott, Christine Stirling, Ben Schüz, and Andrew Robinson. 2016. 'Caring for the Carer: A Systematic Review of Pure Technology-based Cognitive Behavioural Therapy (TB-CBT) Interventions for Dementia Carers.' *Aging & Mental Health* 20 (8): 793–803.

Shaji, K. Sivaraman, K. Smitha, K. Praveen Lal, and Martin J. Prince. 2003. 'Caregivers of People with Alzheimer's Disease: A Qualitative Study from the Indian 10/66 Dementia Research Network.' *International Journal of Geriatric Psychiatry* 18 (1): 1–6.

Sussman, R. J. 1998. 'Online Counselling.' *Counselling Today* 40: 8–20.

Swinton, Jonathan J., W. David Robinson, and Richard J. Bischoff. 2009. 'Telehealth and Rural Depression: Physician and Patient Perspectives.' *Families, Systems, & Health* 27 (2): 172.

Wang, Jing, Lily Dongxia Xiao, Xiaomei Li, Anita De Bellis, and Shahid Ullah. 2015. 'Caregiver Distress and Associated Factors in Dementia Care in the Community Setting in China.' *Geriatric Nursing* 36 (5): 348–354.

World Health Organization. 2012. 'Dementia Cases Set to Triple by 2050 but Still Largely Ignored.' Available at: https://www.who.int/mediacentre/news/releases/2012/dementia_20120411/en/ (accessed on 17 December 2019).

Yashaswini, R., and Prema K. S. Rao. 2018. 'Tele Speech-Language Pathology and Audiology in India: A Short Report.' *Journal of the International Society for Telemedicine and eHealth* 6 e19-1.

Computer-assisted Programs for Children with Specific Learning Disorder

Implications and Challenges

Vimala Jayakrishna Kasturi and Sanjeev Kumar Gupta

INTRODUCTION

Children, during their early developmental period, first learn to understand the spoken language and then to speak. During their school years, they learn to read, write and solve arithmetic as per their age and cognitive ability. However, every child would not be able to learn as per their age and ability. Across the globe, children with a specific learning disorder (SLD) are struggling to excel in academic life. The *Diagnostic and Statistical Manual of Mental Disorders* (American Psychiatric Association 2013) considers an SLD to be 'a type of Neurodevelopmental Disorder that impedes the ability to learn or use specific academic skills (e.g., reading, writing, or arithmetic), which are the foundations for other academic learning'. Children with SLDs (CwSLDs) often face difficulties in fluent word recognition and decoding skills (Lyon, Shaywitz and Shaywitz 2003). About 5–10 per cent of the population is affected by developmental dyslexia (Peterson and Pennington 2015; Shaywitz et al. 1990). Although scanty, in the Indian context, 2–18 per cent incidences of dyslexia in primary school children, 14 per cent of dysgraphia and 5.5 per cent of dyscalculia are reported (Mittal et al. 1977; Ramaa and Gowramma 2002; Shah, Khanna and Pinto 1981).

Among the several theories that have tried to explain the deficits in SLDs, the most common ones are 'general auditory' (Baldeweg et al. 1999; Farmer and Klein 1995; Reed 1989; Tallal 1980), 'visual' (Livingstone and Hubel 1988; Lovegrove et al. 1980; Stein and Walsh 1997), 'motor impairments' (Nicolson and Fawcett 1990; Rudel 1985; Wolff, Michel and Ovrut 1990) and 'phonological processing deficit hypothesis' (Bradley and Bryant 1983; Ramus et al. 2003)'. Lachmann and van Leeuwen (2014) proposed that difficulties in learning grapheme–phoneme associations are experienced by CwSLDs, and that these skills remain suboptimal even after they are acquired. Owing to these deficits, CwSLDs expend more energy than typical children do in reading and also underperform at reading fluently (Sprenger-Charolles, Colé and Serniclaes 2013; Vaessen and Blomert 2010). Grapho-phonemic training has been the focus of many intervention studies to enable or improve reading skills in CwSLDs.

Educational, technical and medical intervention to help students with SLDs were proposed by Alwell and Cobb (2009). Brown (2002) recommended the use of multimedia to improve the accessibility to the learning environment. He suggested presenting graphic or auditory forms along with text to minimize the difficulties of recognizing or confusing between letters and familiar words. Providing auditory forms as supplements to texts was thought to help CwSLDs form links between graphemes and phonemes of new words. Gaining popularity in the recent times, the use of computer-assisted technology and multimedia or telerehabilitation (TR) is being researched to establish their efficacy in the treatment of SLDs.

Currently, the TR applications encompass four main health care areas: (a) control at a distance of clients and rehabilitative services, (b) computer-assisted rehabilitation exercises (physical and cognitive), (c) communication among clients, doctors and caregivers, and (d) distance training either for clients or for rehabilitation personnel. TR services are delivered to adults and children by a broad range of professionals that may include, but are not limited to, psychologists, speech–language pathologists, audiologists, physical therapists, occupational therapists, rehabilitation physicians and nurses, rehabilitation engineers, assistive technologists, and dieticians, as other personnel such as paraprofessionals, family members and caregivers may assist during TR sessions. Software-based teletreatment, a type of computer-assisted rehabilitation, is core to the process of TR as it permits interaction between the instructor and the person through long distance in an asynchronous manner (Marzano and Pellegrino 2017).

The current review aimed at assimilating and organizing available information on educational or rehabilitation technology or TR for SLDs and providing educators and therapists with evidence-based data for the use of technological applications for the rehabilitation of CwSLDs. The objective of the study was to provide an overview of the available educational or TR applications for SLDs through an extensive research synthesis for better implementation of evidence-based technology.

METHOD

The current narrative review about computer-assisted programs for SLDs was conducted through an Internet search of databases using keywords such as computerized instruction, computer-based instruction, computer-directed instruction, computer-mediated instruction, TR applications, apps, dyslexia, learning disorder and treatment. Various types of resources such as journal articles, review articles, books, theses and dissertations were reviewed over a period of one year (Figure 11.1). Following this, a set of seven specific computer-assisted programs or

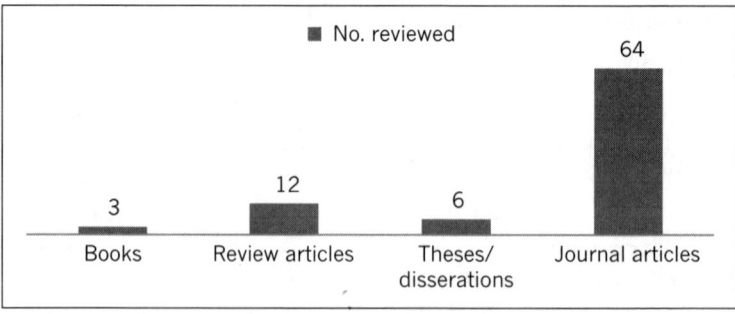

Figure 11.1 *Number and Type of Resources Reviewed*

multimedia applications were identified, which were frequently occurring in the literature search from a set of 85 resources using search engines such as Google Scholar, PubMed and ScienceDirect, which covered online journals. After carefully scrutinizing the abstracts of articles that showed up on the Internet search, only those that were related to the frequently occurring computer-assisted programs or multimedia applications were shortlisted for the review.

The articles which essentially aimed at treatment or rehabilitation using a certain technological application were selected after reading the abstract. A thorough read of the full-length articles related to these frequently occurring computer-assisted programs or multimedia applications was done to understand and evaluate various aspects of the program such as specific details of the developed program, the areas or skills remediated by the program, population or age group of the target, and efficacy or evidence supporting or nullifying the results. No statistical procedures were employed. However, a subjective critical analysis was employed to understand the factors related to the usage of computer-assisted technology and their efficacy.

RESEARCH REVIEW, CHALLENGES AND ISSUES

A Brief History

The use of computers in teaching has been prevalent since the 1920s. However, the use of computers has branched to cover a wide variety of students as well as subjects over time. Three eras delineate the evolution of the use of computers in education: (a) 1920s–1950s (b) 1950s–1980s and (c) 1980s–date. One of the first uses of computers was to deliver simple drill-and-practice exercises, where immediate feedback would be received regarding the answers in the educational set-up between the 1920s and the 1950s. It was thought that it would ease the burden of teachers in terms of grading assignments and help them focus on making the teaching process more inspirational and thought stimulating. Although primarily developed for military operations (Molnar 1997), the ability of computer systems such as MARK I and ENIAC to rapidly automate mathematical functions made them extremely useful for educational purposes (Weik 1964). Between the

1950s and the 1980s, there was a surge in the making of a number of systems that were based on the principles of instructional programming. One of the drill-and-practice methods for mathematics which could be modified for each of the students called Programmed Logic for Automatic Teaching Operations (PLATO) was implemented in 1959. From the 1980s onwards, a boom in the mass production of computers and growth of the World Wide Web and the Internet were prominent and led to the increased use of computers in education systems. As a parallel development that took place in the modern era with faster computers and the World Wide Web coming into existence, it came to the notice of many researchers that the look-and-say method that was being used was not successful with all the students, and thus the potential failure of the American education system was realized. Hence, phonics-based programs started gaining popularity. However, the struggle to learn to read and write could not be eased with the changing methods either. The need for research towards finding effective strategies for classroom teaching was much felt (Alexander and Fox 2004).

In the 1990s, with the emergence of newer technology, computer-assisted methods were beginning to become a part of the teaching strategies, and their effectiveness was being established. Very many titles such as computerized instruction, computer-based instruction, computer-directed instruction and computer-mediated instruction have all been used to describe the process of using computers to assist in teaching students. Despite the varied nomenclature, each of these titles refers to the basic idea of using computers to assist in the instruction of students. As described by Frenzel (1980), computer-assisted instruction (CAI) is 'the process by which written and visual information is presented in a logical sequence to a student by a computer'. Reducing the requirement of in-person training, CAI is beneficial especially because it can provide immediate feedback as well as continually adjust the material being (Baroody 1986; Mastropieri, Bakken and Scruggs 1991).

Effectiveness of CAI

A meta-analysis of 26 research studies, which examined the effectiveness of CAI in different subject areas, conducted from 1984 to 1995 was carried out by Chirstmann, Badgett and Lucking (1997). Students from secondary schools were placed into three groups: (a) those who received only traditional lecture-style instruction, (b) those who received traditional instruction that was augmented with CAI and (c) those who received only CAI instruction. The gains on standardized tests were observed to be higher for those students who received exposure to CAI in the classroom, either alone or integrated into traditional lecture-style instruction, than those who received only traditional lecture-style instruction. The researchers also stated that since CAI could automatically adjust to each student's learning pace, it increased individual learning time, thereby having an overall long-term positive effect. Effectiveness of the basic skills/computer education program in the 1991–1992 school years was examined by Mann et al. (1999) in West Virginia. Over 900 fifth graders were assessed for spelling, vocabulary, reading and mathematics to examine the effectiveness of the program in teaching. An increase in the score of the Stanford 9 test in the mentioned areas was witnessed for students who received CAI. In addition, students with SLDs achieved the greatest gains on their test scores. Li (2002) studied the impact of CAI on the language and collaboration skills using the new technology in a variety of academic settings. He found that students' interaction increased using CAI and thus their achievement. Each of these studies provided a positive overall picture of using CAI in the classroom. However, they generally failed to isolate the effectiveness of this method of instruction for students with SLDs.

CAI and Children with Reading Disorder

For children with a reading disorder, CAI procedures that remediated accuracy and speed of response were used by Fiedorowicz (1986). Skills like those of decoding and phonetic knowledge were targeted. When given remediation using computers, significant gains in the speed and accuracy on single-syllable, phonetically regular words were reported by Jones, Torgesen and Sexton (1987). This study also showed a generalization of the treatment to unpractised words while reading. Yet another study reported that CAI practice transferred to an oral reading of words in print when two- and three-syllable words were practised in a multiple-choice format by students with a reading disorder (Torgesen et al. 1988). Furthermore, numerous reading skills such as vocabulary (Johnson, Gersten and Carnine 1987), comprehension (VanDen Meiracker 1987) and reading engagement (Harper and Ewing 1986) have been successfully remediated by CAI. Among the advantages that CAI has to offer, word recognition (Wong 1991), one-to-one practice within classrooms while minimizing the supervisory time by the teacher and the scope for immediate correction of responses owing to the immediate feedback (Torgesen et al. 1988) are a few. CAI has also been employed to remediate phonological awareness skills in children with autism (Heimann et al. 1995; Tjus, Heimann and Nelson 1998). In addition, Williams et al. (2002) reported better reading performance on CAI format of presentation than traditional presentation in a book for students with autism as the attention span was noted to be higher for the CAI format of presentation through a computer. For students with impaired speech and accompanying physical disabilities and autism, there is only scanty research. While these studies are useful for comparing different types of CAI programs, they are not appropriate for answering the question of whether CAI was as effective as other methods of instruction that did not utilize computers.

Among the articles that were published on treatment using a certain technological program which were considered for the current review, there were two articles on Fast ForWord, seven on Success for All (SFA), nine on READ 180, seven on Great Leaps Reading, one on Earobics and one on Read, Write & Type (RWT) as depicted in Figure 11.2. These articles also included review articles published along the same lines of research.

Fast ForWord

Fast ForWord® is a computer-based reading program, developed by Scientific Learning Corporation to develop and strengthen the cognitive skills necessary for successful reading and learning by the use of audiovisual games (Strong et al. 2011). The program is recommended to be used 30–100 minutes a day, 5 days a week, for 4–16 weeks and includes 3 series. To review the effectiveness of this program, one review article and two journal articles were selected. From this

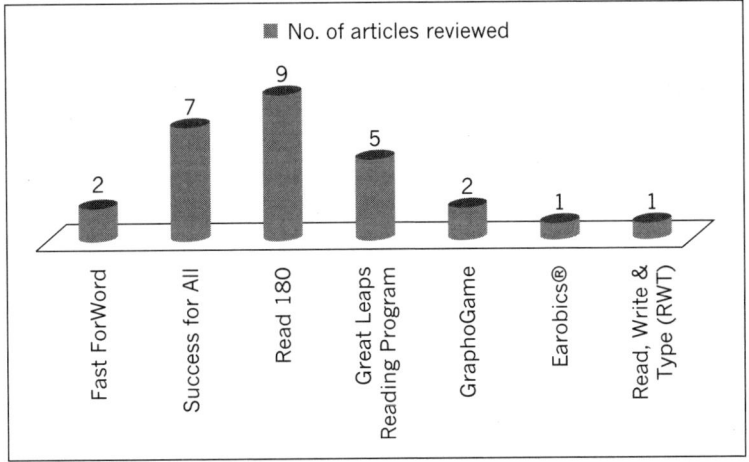

Figure 11.2 *Number of Articles Reviewed for Each of the Seven Specific Programs Discussed*

review, nine studies were found to have positive outcomes, two studies reported negative outcomes and the other studies were inconclusive as they did not meet the required research standards (Table 11.1; Figure 11.3).

Success for All

In the SFA (Madden 1991) reading program, a combination of multimedia presentation and computer-assisted tutoring was used to create a novel method of reading instruction. On reviewing the published literature on this software, two school-level implementation studies reported positive outcomes (Table 11.1; Figure 11.3).

READ 180

Created by Scholastic Corporation, READ 180 is a program for reading remediation for students of Grades 4–12 whose reading skills are at least 2 years below their grade level. It makes use of adaptive technology to design appropriate curriculum, instruction, assessment and professional development to remediate the reading abilities of students who struggle to read. It is available in three stages, each

Table 11.1 Specific Computer-assisted Programs/Applications for Remediation of Reading

Author/Publisher	Population/Sample/Studies	Domain	Type of Evidence
Fast ForWord			
Strong et al. (2011)	Reviewing 79 relevant studies; meta-analysis study	Literacy skills; oral language	1 negative evidence
Given, Wasserman, Chare, Beattie and Eden (2008)	65 middle school students	Reading domain	1 negative evidence
What Works Clearinghouse review (henceforth referred to as WWC, updated in March 2013)	342 studies that reported the effects of Fast ForWord	Alphabet, reading fluency and comprehension	9 positive evidences; statistically significant 317 out of scope for review
Success for All (SFA)			
Tracey, Chambers, Slavin, Hanley and Cheung (2014)	18 SFA schools across England and 18 control schools, matched on prior achievement and demographics	Phonics; word-level reading	1 positive evidence; statistically significant
Smith, Ross and Casey (1996)	Participants were SFA and control-school primary-grade students (K-2) at four sites implementing SFA	Reading	1 positive evidence; statistically significant
READ 180			
Kim, Capotosto, Harry and Fitzgerald (2011)	312 students (155 programs, 157 control)	General reading; comprehension	1 positive evidence; statistically significant

WWC (2010)	56 studies of READ 180® for students with learning disabilities that were published or released between 1989 and 2009	Reading	2 positive evidences; statistically not significant
			54 out of scope for review
WWC (2009a)	WWC reviewed 101 studies on READ 180 for adolescent learners	Reading	7 positive evidences; statistically significant
			94 out of scope for review
Kim et al. (2006)	A total of 294 children in Grades 4–6 were randomly assigned to READ 180 or a district after-school programme	Reading	1 negative evidence
Kim, Capotosto, Harry and Fitzgerald (2011)	19 middle schools	Reading	1 positive evidence; statistically significant
Gober (2014)	170 seventh- and 207 eighth-grade English language learners enrolled in READ180 and traditional communication arts	Reading	1 positive evidence; statistically significant

Great Leaps Reading Program (GLRP)

Mercer, Campbell, Miller, Mercer and Lane (2000)	49 middle school students with learning disabilities	Reading	1 positive evidence; statistically significant
Haselden and Webster (2011)	Three participants with documented disabilities in the area of reading	Reading	1 positive evidence; statistically significant
Hacker (2008)	Two English as second language siblings, a third-grader and a fourth-grader were selected for this classroom study	Oral reading	1 positive evidence; statistically significant

(Table 11.1 Continued)

(Table 11.1 Continued)

Author/Publisher	Population/Sample/Studies	Domain	Type of Evidence
GraphoGame			
Mönkkönen et al. (2014)	Kindergarten children played GraphoGame Reading (n = 58) and others (n = 52) played the GraphoGame Math. Nonplaying controls were 41	Reading and letter knowledge	1 positive evidence; statistically significant
Saine, Lerkkanen, Ahonen, Tolvanen and Lyytinen (2011)	Two cohorts of children from four schools from the same district (n = 166) were followed	Reading	1 positive evidence; statistically significant
Brem et al. (2010)	German-speaking kindergarten children (n = 32; 6–7 years of age) played the game	Reading	1 positive evidence; statistically significant
Kyle, Kujala, Richardson, Lyytinen and Goswami (2013)	English-speaking second-graders (6- to 7-year-olds) in the United Kingdom	Rhyme production and phonics	1 positive evidence; statistically significant
Earobics®			
WWC (2009b)	Reviewed 28 studies	Alphabetics reading fluency	4 positive evidences; statistically significant
			24 out of scope for review
Read, Write & Type (RWT)			
Torgesen, Wagner, Rashotte and Herron (2018)	150 low-achieving first-grade students in 5 elementary schools	Alphabetics	1 positive evidence; statistically significant
WWC (2009c)			2 negative evidences
		Comprehension	2 negative evidences

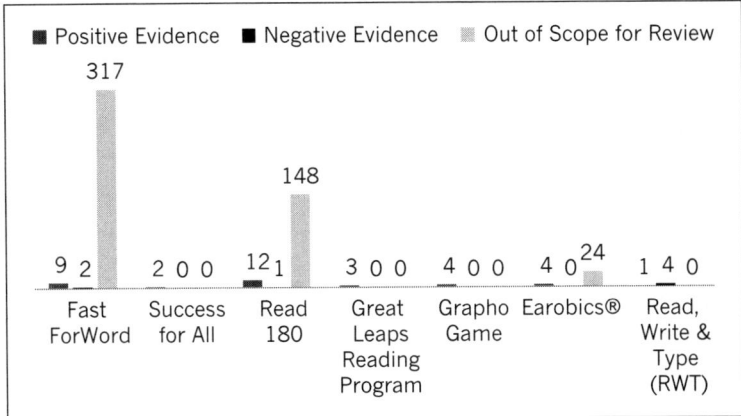

Figure 11.3 *Proportions of Evidence for Each of the Seven Reviewed Programs*

with rigorous, age-appropriate content: (a) Stage A (Grades 4–6), (b) Stage B (Grades 6–8) and (c) Stage C (Grades 9 and above). A total of 12 studies reported positive outcomes and 1 negative, and 148 studies were out of the scope for review for this program when a total of 2 review articles and 4 independent journal articles were reviewed (Table 11.1; Figure 11.3).

Great Leaps Reading

Great Leaps Reading program was developed to supplement the reading instructions of students with reading difficulties to be used in conjunction with the curriculum currently being implemented for a student with its primary focus on fluency (Campbell 1994). The studies that reported positive outcomes of using this program were three in number when a review of three independent journal articles was carried out (Table 11.1; Figure 11.3).

GraphoGame

GraphoGame, a new computerized phonics training program, was designed to strengthen the links between orthographic and phonological encodings (for a review, see Richardson and Lyytinen 2014).

A simultaneous and repeated presentation of grapheme–phoneme correspondences (first in isolation, then included in syllables, and afterwards in words) to fluency training with words and sentences is used in this method. GraphoGame is recommended to be used as a preventive help and as support but not as a replacement for traditional teaching. The method is meant to be used as a support tool for learning. It is not a replacement of teaching, but it rather provides preventive help. Four studies reported positive outcomes of using this program in the research review done (Table 11.1; Figure 11.3).

Earobics®

Developed in 1995, Earobics®, a computer-assisted training program that aims to improve reading skills by remediating skills such as sound perception, memory and phonological awareness (Diehl 1999; Morrison 1998), is distributed by Houghton Mifflin Harcourt Learning Technology. Comprising of numerous tasks such as phoneme identification and discrimination and rhyme judgements, this program has been widely used in American schools for teaching reading skills to children with language learning difficulties. The studies that reported positive outcomes of using this program were four in number when a review of What Works Clearinghouse (WWC) report published in 2007 was carried out, while there were 24 studies that were considered as being out of scope for review as they did not meet the WWC standards (Table 11.1; Figure 11.3).

Read, Write & Type

RWT is a software program developed by Dr Jeannine Herron and Dr Leslie Grimm and distributed by Talking Fingers Inc. for reading remediation. With the emphasis on writing and as a way to learn to read, this program was developed for 6- to 9-year-old students who are just beginning to read and for children who face difficulties in learning to read and write. The RWT program is based on the premise that directly teaching students the spellings of phonemes and using that knowledge to support spelling and writing activities may have unique advantages in helping students master the alphabetic principle (Herron 2008). Among the studies reviewed, one reported the positive

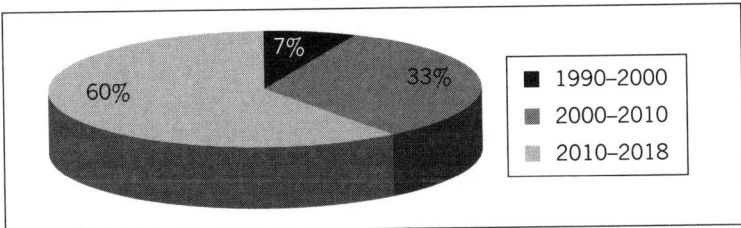

Figure 11.4 *Year-Wise Split of Articles Published on the Usage of Technology for Rehabilitation of SLDs*

effects of using this program, while four reported no positive outcomes (Table 11.1; Figure 11.3).

In summary, it was found that 6 articles were published in the 1990s, 28 articles in the 2000s and 51 articles between 2001 and 2017 (Figure 11.4).

In total, 34 studies across various technological programs had positive effects after usage of the technological program, and 178 studies did not meet standards in terms of appropriate research designs, statistically significant results and appropriate methods of implementing the training (Table 11.1; Figure 11.3). Most commonly, the domains of literacy skills, alphabetics, oral language, reading fluency, reading and reading comprehension were remediated by most of the programs (Figure 11.5). Among the various skills that different programs targeted, reading,

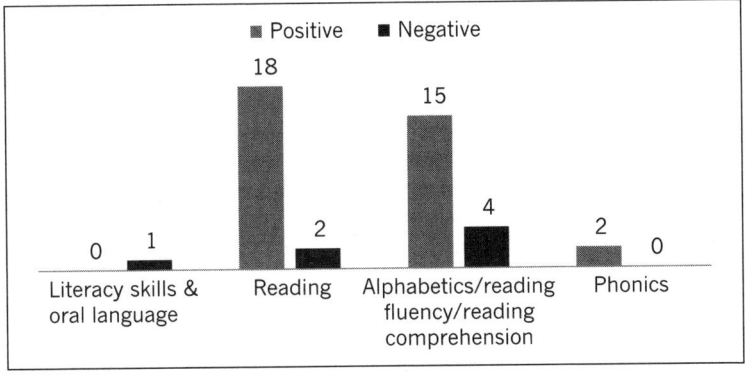

Figure 11.5 *Skills Which Evidenced Positive Effects across Seven Reviewed Programmes*

reading fluency, alphabetics and reading comprehension evidenced maximum gains according to the current review (Figure 11.5).

STRENGTHS AND WEAKNESSES OF COMPUTER-ASSISTED PROGRAMS

The usage of CAI has evolved over the years. Potential benefits that accompany the use of CAI are self-paced learning, self-directed learning, reduction in supervision time by the teachers, provision for repeated practice and immediate feedback. Computers are considered to have an encouraging effect on learning as they provide a stimulating environment and provide enthusiasm (Meskill and Mossop 1997). For a reticent student who is afraid to make mistakes in a classroom situation, CAI may prove to be of help (Chun 1994; Meskill and Swan 1996). The advantage of the gaming format of CAI is that it has both recreational and didactic goals (García, Kloos and Gil 2008). Successful educational games intend to grab the interest of a student, thereby motivating him/her to acquire knowledge (Kast et al. 2011).

Although there are many advantages of using educational technology, certain unplanned side effects must also be foreseen by the instructor. He/she must be cautious in choosing the kind of educational technology that best suits the student in question (Furr, Ragsdale and Horton 2005). One of such downsides of using educational technology is the time and effort required to create resources for instructions using multimedia. It must be understood that the mere use of educational technology by itself will not guarantee learning. By simply providing interesting material for therapy, a structured method of providing intervention using a logical learning hierarchy, immediate feedbacks and many trials for practice, computer-assisted technology may prove to be helpful in remediation. Using CAI is one way for a teacher to differentiate instructions. Students in secondary school classrooms who lack reading skills may struggle to comprehend the written material, and providing effective interventions for struggling readers is difficult when CAI may be one way to address the concerns of teachers who lack the knowledge and skills to teach at-risk students and when the instructional resources needed are not available (Torgesen et al. 2010).

CONCLUSION

A study by DeBell (2005) found that while 91 per cent of typically developing students in a class used computers, only 82 per cent of the CwSLDs did so. A similar finding for the usage of the Internet was reported where over 60 per cent of the typically developing children of a class used the Internet, while less than half of CwSLDs did so. On scrutinizing the reasons for such disparity in usage of computers among CwSLDs and their non-disabled peers, lack of research regarding the effectiveness of CAI programs for students with disorders, especially those with SLDs, and conflicting teacher and student attitude towards using these technologies were noted to be prominent (Barron et al. 2003; Wilson and Notar 2003). When a review was piloted to study the usage of CAI in teaching mathematics to students with SLDs through computerized databases, Internet searches and book reviews, only 23 research studies were found that were completed within the past 25 years. Out of these 23 studies, experimental methods of research were employed in 14 of the studies, single group studies were 4 in number and hybrid approaches were used in 1 study. Failure to isolate the effectiveness of CAI programs was evidenced mainly due to poor experimental design. Of the 23 articles, 5 focused on comparison among different types of CAI rather than studying the efficacy of CAI. On a concluding note, it is recommended that research towards establishing the efficacy of such technology must follow adequate measures to ensure that the quality of research is appropriate. Most research studies go disregarded because of technical issues like weak research design, a fewer number of participants or losing out on reporting the longitudinal effects of the treatment implemented.

Conducting innovative multidisciplinary research in the area of computer-assisted programs or TR will establish the evidence-based practice and rehabilitation methods using technology for the highest benefit of students with SLDs.

REFERENCES

Alexander, Patricia A., and Emily Fox. 2004. 'A Historical Perspective on Reading Research and Practice.' In *Theoretical Models and Processes of Reading*, 5th ed., edited by Norman J. Unrau and Robert B. Ruddell, 33–68. Newark: International Reading Association.

Alwell, Morgen, and Brian Cobb. 2009. 'Functional Life Skills Curricular Interventions for Youth with Disabilities: A Systematic Review.' *Career Development for Exceptional Individuals* 32 (2): 82–93.

American Psychiatric Association. 2013. *Diagnostic and Statistical Manual of Mental Disorders*. 5th ed. Arlington, VA: American Psychiatric Association Publishing.

Baldeweg, Torsten, Alexandra Richardson, Sarah Watkins, Christine Foale, and John Gruzelier. 1999. 'Impaired Auditory Frequency Discrimination in Dyslexia Detected with Mismatch Evoked Potentials.' *Annals of Neurology: Official Journal of the American Neurological Association and the Child Neurology Society* 45 (4): 495–503.

Baroody, Arthur J. 1986. 'The Value of Informal Approaches to Mathematics Instruction and Remediation.' *Arithmetic Teacher* 33 (5): 14–18.

Barron, Ann E., Kate Kemker, Christine Harmes, and Kimberly Kalaydjian. 2003. 'Large-Scale Research Study on Technology in K–12 Schools: Technology Integration as It Relates to the National Technology Standards.' *Journal of Research on Technology in Education* 35 (4): 489–507.

Bradley, Lynette, and Peter E. Bryant. 1983. 'Categorizing Sounds and Learning to Read—A Causal Connection.' *Nature* 301 (5899): 419.

Brem, Silvia, Silvia Bach, Karin Kucian, Janne V. Kujala, Tomi K. Guttorm, Ernst Martin, Heikki Lyytinen, Daniel Brandeis, and Ulla Richardson. 2010. 'Brain Sensitivity to Print Emerges When Children Learn Letter–Speech Sound Correspondences.' *Proceedings of the National Academy of Sciences* 107 (17): 7939–7944.

Brown, Bettina Lankard. 2002. *Generic Skills in Career and Technical Education*. Columbus, OH: ERIC Clearinghouse on Adult, Career, and Vocational Education, Center on Education and Training for Employment, College of Education, Ohio State University.

Campbell, K. U., and C. Mercer. 1994. *Great Leaps Reading*. Micanopy, FL: Diarmuid.

Christmann, Edwin, John Badgett, and Robert Lucking. 1997. 'Microcomputer-based Computer-assisted Instruction within Differing Subject Areas: A Statistical Deduction.' *Journal of Educational Computing Research* 16 (3): 281–296.

Chun, Dorothy M. 1994. 'Using Computer Networking to Facilitate the Acquisition of Interactive Competence.' *System* 22 (1): 17–31.

DeBell, Matthew. 2005. 'Rates of Computer and Internet Use by Children in Nursery School and Students in Kindergarten through Twelfth Grade: 2003.' Issue Brief No. NCES 2005-111. Washington, DC: National Center for Education Statistics.

Diehl, Sylvia Farnsworth. 1999. 'Listen and Learn? A Software Review of Earobics®.' *Language, Speech, and Hearing Services in Schools* 30 (1): 108–116.

Farmer, Mary E., and Raymond M. Klein. 1995. 'The Evidence for a Temporal Processing Deficit Linked to Dyslexia: A Review.' *Psychonomic Bulletin & Review* 2 (4): 460–493.

Fiedorowicz, Christina A. M. 1986. 'Training of Component Reading Skills'. *Annals of Dyslexia* 36 (1): 318–334.

Frenzel, Lou. 1980. 'The Personal Computer: Last Chance for CAI?' *Byte* 5 (7): 86–96.

Furr, Paula F., Ronald Ragsdale, and Steven G. Horton. 2005. 'Technology's Non-neutrality: Past Lessons Can Help Guide Today's Classrooms.' *Education and Information Technologies* 10 (3): 277–287.

García, Raquel M. Crespo, Carlos Delgado Kloos, and Manuel Castro Gil. 2008. 'Game Based Spelling Learning.' Paper presented at 2008 38th Annual Frontiers in Education Conference, S3B–11. IEEE, Saratoga Springs, NY, 22–25 October.

Given, Barbara K., John D. Wasserman, Sharmila A. Chari, Karen Beattie, and Guinevere F. Eden. 2008. 'A Randomized, Controlled Study of Computer-based Intervention in Middle School Struggling Readers.' *Brain and Language* 106 (2): 83–97.

Gober, Carissa. 2014. 'READ 180: Is It an Effective Reading Intervention for English Language Learners?' PhD dissertation. Lindenwood University, Saint Charles, MO.

Hacker, Judith A. 2008. 'Increasing Oral Reading Fluency with Elementary English Language Learners.' Master's thesis. Hamline University, Saint Paul, MN.

Harper, Janice A., and Norma J. Ewing. 1986. 'A Comparison of the Effectiveness of Microcomputer and Workbook Instruction on Reading Comprehension Performance of High Incidence Handicapped Children.' *Educational Technology* 26 (5): 40–45.

Haselden, Polly G., and S. Elizabeth Webster. 2011. 'The Effects of the "Great Leaps Reading Program" on Students with Severe Reading Disabilities as a Secondary Reading Intervention in an Impoverished Setting.' Available at: https://pdfs. semanticscholar.org/1490/9c97d1914039c65ac4fee5a54f41b4c9eb20. pdf?_ga=2.208369232.359558796.1577425225-2100263851.1537947654 (accessed on 27 December 2019).

Heimann, Mikael, Keith E. Nelson, Tomas Tjus, and Christopher Gillberg. 1995. 'Increasing Reading and Communication Skills in Children with Autism through an Interactive Multimedia Computer Program.' *Journal of Autism and Developmental Disorders* 25 (5): 459–480.

Herron, Jeannine. 2008. 'Why Phonics Teaching Must Change.' *Educational Leadership* 66 (1): 77–81.

Johnson, Gary, Russell Gersten, and Douglas Carnine. 1987. 'Effects of Instructional Design Variables on Vocabulary Acquisition of LD Students: A Study of Computer-assisted Instruction.' *Journal of Learning Disabilities* 20 (4): 206–213.

Jones, Kathryn M., Joseph K. Torgesen, and Molly A. Sexton 1987.. 'Using Computer-guided Practice to Increase Decoding Fluency in Learning Disabled Children: A Study Using the Hint and Hunt I Program.' *Journal of Learning Disabilities* 20 (2): 122–128.

Kast, Monika, Gian-Marco Baschera, Markus Gross, Lutz Jäncke, and Martin Meyer. 2011. 'Computer-based Learning of Spelling Skills in Children with and without Dyslexia.' *Annals of Dyslexia* 61 (2): 177–200.

Kim, Ae-Hwa, Sharon Vaughn, Janette K. Klingner, Althea L. Woodruff, Colleen Klein Reutebuch, and Kamiar Kouzekanani. 2006. 'Improving the Reading Comprehension of Middle School Students with Disabilities through Computer-assisted Collaborative Strategic Reading.' *Remedial and Special Education* 27 (4): 235–249.

Kim, James S., Lauren Capotosto, Ardice Hartry, and Robert Fitzgerald. 2011. 'Can a Mixed-Method Literacy Intervention Improve the Reading Achievement of Low-performing Elementary School Students in an After-School Program? Results from a Randomized Controlled Trial of READ 180 Enterprise.' *Educational Evaluation and Policy Analysis* 33 (2): 183–201.

Kyle, Fiona, Janne Kujala, Ulla Richardson, Heikki Lyytinen, and Usha Goswami. 2013. 'Assessing the Effectiveness of Two Theoretically Motivated Computer-assisted Reading Interventions in the United Kingdom: GG Rime and GG Phoneme.' *Reading Research Quarterly* 48 (1): 61–76.

Lachmann, Thomas, and Cees van Leeuwen. 2014. 'Reading as Functional Coordination: Not Recycling but a Novel Synthesis.' *Frontiers in Psychology* 5: 1046.

Li, Qing. 2002. 'Exploration of Collaborative Learning and Communication in an Educational Environment Using Computer-mediated Communication.' *Journal of Research on Technology in Education* 34 (4): 503–516.

Livingstone, Margaret, and David Hubel. 1988. 'Segregation of Form, Color, Movement, and Depth: Anatomy, Physiology, and Perception.' *Science* 240 (4853): 740–749.

Lovegrove, William J., Alison Bowling, D. Badcock, and Mary Blackwood. 1980. 'Specific Reading Disability: Differences in Contrast Sensitivity as a Function of Spatial Frequency.' *Science* 210 (4468): 439–440.

Lyon, G. Reid, Sally E. Shaywitz, and Bennett A. Shaywitz. 2003. 'A Definition of Dyslexia.' *Annals of Dyslexia* 53 (1): 1–14.

Madden, Nancy A. 1991. *Success for All: Multi-year Effects of a Schoolwide Elementary Restructuring Program.* Report No. 18. Baltimore, MD: Center for Research on Effective Schooling for Disadvantaged Students.

Mann, Dale, Charol Shakeshaft, Jonathan D. Becker, and Robert Kottkamp. 1999. 'West Virginia Story: Achievement Gains from a Statewide Comprehensive Instructional Technology Program.' Available at: https://pdfs.semantic-scholar.org/d5e1/ed74a879b7cc4fbcfdfb6c9502bf29e641d9.pdf (accessed on 27 December 2019).

Marzano, Gilberto, and Anna Pellegrino. 2017. 'Towards the Organization of Telerehabilitation Services.' *JOJ Nurse & Health Care* 1 (3): 555562.

Mastropieri, Margo A., Jeffrey P. Bakken, and Thomas E. Scruggs. 1991. 'Mathematics Instruction for Individuals with Mental Retardation: A Perspective and Research Synthesis.' *Education and Training in Mental Retardation* 26 (2): 115–129.

Mercer, Cecil D., Kenneth U. Campbell, M. David Miller, Kenneth D. Mercer, and Holly B. Lane. 2000. 'Effects of a Reading Fluency Intervention for Middle Schoolers with Specific Learning Disabilities.' *Learning Disabilities Research & Practice* 15 (4): 179–189.

Meskill, Carla, and Jonathan Mossop. 1997. *Technologies Use with ESL Learners in New York State: Preliminary Report.* Report Series 3.13. Albany, NY: National Research Center on English Learning & Achievement.

Meskill, Carla, and Karen Swan. 1996. 'Roles for Multimedia in the Response-based Literature Classroom.' *Journal of Educational Computing Research* 15 (3): 217–239.

Mittal, S. K., I. Zaidi, N. Puri, S. Duggal, B. Rath, and S. K. Bhargava. 1977. 'Communication Disabilities: Emerging Problems of Childhood.' *Indian Pediatrics* 14 (10): 811–815.

Molnar, Andrew. 1997. 'Computers in Education: A Brief History.' *The Journal* 24 (11): 63–68.

Mönkkönen, A., S. Bach, S. Brem, J. Erskine, J. Kujala, G. Willems, and U. Richardson. 2014. 'Technology Enhanced Training of Basic Decoding Skills in Preschool Age Children.' Manuscript in preparation.

Morrison, S. 1998. 'Earobics Pro (1997).' *Child Language Teaching and Therapy* 14: 279–284.

Nicolson, Roderick I., and Angela J. Fawcett. 1990. 'Automaticity: A New Framework for Dyslexia Research?' *Cognition* 35 (2): 159–182.

Peterson, Robin L., and Bruce F. Pennington. 2015. 'Developmental Dyslexia.' *Annual Review of Clinical Psychology* 11: 283–307.

Ramaa, S., and I. P. Gowramma. 2002. 'A Systematic Procedure for Identifying and Classifying Children with Dyscalculia among Primary School Children in India.' *Dyslexia* 8 (2): 67–85.

Ramus, Franck, Stuart Rosen, Steven C. Dakin, Brian L. Day, Juan M. Castellote, Sarah White, and Uta Frith. 2003. 'Theories of Developmental Dyslexia: Insights from a Multiple Case Study of Dyslexic Adults.' *Brain* 126 (4): 841–865.

Reed, Marjorie A. 1989. 'Speech Perception and the Discrimination of Brief Auditory Cues in Reading Disabled Children.' *Journal of Experimental Child Psychology* 48 (2): 270–292.

Richardson, Ulla, and Heikki Lyytinen. 2014. 'The GraphoGame Method: The Theoretical and Methodological Background of the Technology-enhanced Learning Environment for Learning to Read.' *Human Technology* 10 (1): 39–60.

Rudel, R. G. 1985. 'The Definition of Dyslexia: Language and Motor Deficits.' In *Dyslexia: A Neuroscientific Approach to Clinical Evaluation*, edited by F. H. Duffy and N. Geschwind, 33–53. Boston, MA: Little Brown.

Saine, Nina L., Marja-Kristiina Lerkkanen, Timo Ahonen, Asko Tolvanen, and Heikki Lyytinen. 2011. 'Computer-assisted Remedial Reading Intervention for School Beginners at Risk for Reading Disability.' *Child Development* 82 (3): 1013–1028.

Shah, B. P., S. A. Khanna, and N. Pinto. 1981. 'Detection of Learning Disabilities in School Children.' *The Indian Journal of Pediatrics* 48 (6): 767–771.

Shaywitz, Sally E., Bennett A. Shaywitz, Jack M. Fletcher, and Michael D. Escobar. 1990. 'Prevalence of Reading Disability in Boys and Girls: Results of the Connecticut Longitudinal Study.' *JAMA* 264 (8): 998–1002.

Smith, Lana J., Steven M. Ross, and Jason Casey. 1996. 'Multi-site Comparison of the Effects of Success for All on Reading Achievement.' *Journal of Literacy Research* 28 (3): 329–353.

Sprenger-Charolles, Liliane, Pascale Colé, and Willy Serniclaes. 2013. *Reading Acquisition and Developmental Dyslexia*. Hove: Psychology Press.

Stein, John, and Vincent Walsh. 1997. 'To See but Not to Read; the Magnocellular Theory of Dyslexia.' *Trends in Neurosciences* 20 (4): 147–152.

Strong, Gemma K., Carole J. Torgerson, David Torgerson, and Charles Hulme. 2011. 'A Systematic Meta-analytic Review of Evidence for the Effectiveness of the "Fast ForWord" Language Intervention Program.' *Journal of Child Psychology and Psychiatry* 52 (3): 224–235.

Tallal, Paula. 1980. 'Auditory Temporal Perception, Phonics, and Reading Disabilities in Children.' *Brain and Language* 9 (2): 182–198.

Tjus, Tomas, Mikael Heimann, and Keith E. Nelson. 1998. 'Gains in Literacy through the Use of a Specially Developed Multimedia Computer Strategy: Positive Findings from 13 Children with Autism.' *Autism* 2 (2): 139–156.

Torgesen, Joseph K., Mary D. Waters, Andrew L. Cohen, and Jeffery L. Torgesen. 1988. 'Improving Sight-Word Recognition Skills in LD Children: An Evaluation of Three Computer Program Variations.' *Learning Disability Quarterly* 11 (2): 125–132.

Torgesen, Joseph K., Richard K. Wagner, Carol A. Rashotte, and Jeannine Herron. 2018. *Summary of Outcomes from First Grade Study with 'Read, Write, and Type' and 'Auditory Discrimination in Depth' Instruction and Software with At-Risk Children*. FCRR Technical Report No. 2. Tallahassee, FL: Florida Center for Reading Research.

Torgesen, Joseph K., Richard K. Wagner, Carol A. Rashotte, Jeannine Herron, and Patricia Lindamood. 2010. 'Computer-assisted Instruction to Prevent Early Reading Difficulties in Students at Risk for Dyslexia: Outcomes from Two Instructional Approaches.' *Annals of Dyslexia* 60 (1): 40–56.

Tracey, Louise, Bette Chambers, Robert E. Slavin, Pam Hanley, and Alan Cheung. 2014. 'Success for All in England: Results from the Third Year of a National Evaluation.' *SAGE Open* 4 (3). doi:10.1177/2158244014547031

Vaessen, Anniek, and Leo Blomert. 2010. 'Long-Term Cognitive Dynamics of Fluent Reading Development.' *Journal of Experimental Child Psychology* 105 (3): 213–231.

VanDen Meiracker, Maud. 1987. 'Effectiveness of Teacher-based versus Computer-based Instruction on Reading Comprehension of Subtypes of Learning Disabled Children.' *Dissertation Abstract International* 47 (9-A): 3398–3399.

Weik, Martin H. 1964. *A Fourth Survey of Domestic Electronic Digital Computing Systems*. Report No. 1227. Aberdeen, MD: Ballistic Research Laboratory.

Williams, Christine, Barry Wright, Gillian Callaghan, and Brian Coughlan. 2002. 'Do Children with Autism Learn to Read More Readily by Computer-assisted Instruction or Traditional Book Methods? A Pilot Study.' *Autism* 6 (1): 71–91.

Wilson, Janell, and Charles Notar. 2003. 'Use of Computers by Secondary Teachers: A Report from a University Service Area.' *Education* 123 (4): 695.

Wolff, Peter H., George F. Michel, and Marsha Ovrut. 1990. 'Rate Variables and Automatized Naming in Developmental Dyslexia.' *Brain and Language* 39 (4): 556–575.

Wong, Bernice Y. L. 1991. 'The Relevance of Metacognition to Learning Disabilities.' In *Learning about Learning Disabilities*, 231–258. San Diego, CA: Elsevier Academic Press.

What Works Claringhouse. 2009a. *Earobics®*. WWC Intervention Report. Washington, DC: Institute of Education Sciences, United States Department of Education.

———. 2009b. *READ 180®*. WWC Intervention Report. Washington, DC: Institute of Education Sciences, United States Department of Education.

———. 2009c. *Read, Write, and Type™*. WWC Intervention Report. Washington, DC: Institute of Education Sciences, United States Department of Education.

———. 2010. *READ 180®*. WWC Intervention Report. Washington, DC: Institute of Education Sciences, United States Department of Education.

———. 2013. *Fast ForWord®*. WWC Intervention Report. Washington: Institute of Education Sciences, United States Department of Education.

Telerehabilitation in Substance Use Disorder

12

Tanu Gupta and Kartik Singhai

INTRODUCTION

Substance use disorders (SUD) include a group of chronic, enduring and relapsing disorders which form a major chunk of the mental disorder burden in our country. It encompasses the consumption of various drugs such as alcohol, cannabis, hallucinogens, inhalants, opioids, hypnotics, caffeine, anxiolytics and tobacco etc. The essential feature of SUD is the consistent use of the substance irrespective of problems encountered due to substance, resulting in a collection of cognitive, behavioural and physiological symptoms. There is concurrent neglect of routine roles and responsibilities. DSM–5 defines features to diagnose SUD as the presence of increased craving, lack of control, tolerance, risky use despite the evident social impairment (Diagnostic and Statistical Manual of Mental Disorders; DSM–5®; American Psychiatric Association, n.d.).

PREVALENCE RATE

The overall prevalence for any current substance use disorder was found to be 22.7 per cent as per the recently conducted National Mental Health Survey (NMHS) 2015–2016 (Murthy 2017). The prevalence rate cited more in rural areas (24.1%) followed by the urban non-metro (20.3%) and urban metro areas (18.3%). It was highest, that is, 29.4 per cent in the 50–59 years age group with higher prevalence rates in males compared to females (35.7%) (Murthy 2017).

One-fourth respondents reported current tobacco use and 83.6 per cent fulfil the criteria of tobacco use disorder. Here also, the prevalence was predominant in males (1.1%) compared to females (0.1%).

Urbanization and industrialization seem to be the driving factors towards experimental use of the substance of abuse among the youth. The NMHS also reported a significant treatment gap for various mental disorders, which for SUD was 90 per cent. The treatment gap for tobacco was 91.8 per cent compared to 86.3 per cent in alcohol use disorders (AUDs) and 72.9 per cent for other drug use disorders. Mbua et al. (2008) found the estimate of the treatment gap in lower-middle income countries as 56/100.

THE RATIONALE FOR THE CHAPTER

The prevalence rates of SUD are ever-increasing as stated above. The problem with SUD management is its nature of frequent lapses and relapses that make the condition chronic and increases the burden of care. The major reason for relapse is the lack of consistent monitoring on the part of treating doctor and fluctuating motivation from the patient's side. So, with the advent of telehealth (TH) in SUD, the problems can be well addressed and thus, improve the outcome. The chapter aims to disseminate up to date information on the novel technology-assisted psychotherapeutic measures such as text-based cognitive behavioural therapy, transdermal alcohol sensor and others, that have been recently developed worldwide to overcome the obstacles in delivering care to patients with SUD. Further, the chapter shall include discussion on the scope and challenges in providing telerehabilitation (TR) services for substance use disorders.

CURRENT MODES OF TREATMENT

The currently available modes of treatment for substance use disorders largely include pharmacologic agents and non-pharmacological methods.

Pharmacological agents can be broadly defined in two categories: those used for managing the acute withdrawal/detoxification phase and those used for the long-term maintenance/relapse prevention phase. Agents used for the long-term management of AUDs include Naltrexone, Acamprosate and Disulfiram. The choice of the drug depends on different variables such as illness profile, patient profile and the clinician's choice. Similarly, for opioid use disorders, Naltrexone as an anti-craving agent and Buprenorphine or Methadone as maintenance therapy are the available expedients. Along same lines, Bupropion and Varenicline along with Nicotine replacement therapy are used as pharmacological measures for tobacco use disorders. No specific and approved agents are yet available for various SUDs such as cannabis, hallucinogens and psychostimulants. However, the efficacy of some drugs with limited strength of evidence is available and is used worldwide as per the discretion of the treating clinician.

Non-pharmacological measures include various therapies commonly applicable to most SUDs include: motivational enhancement therapy, relapse prevention therapy, cognitive behaviour therapy for individual SUDs, tobacco cessation therapy, family therapy, to name a few.

The reasons for the limited efficacy of the treatment for SUDs are manifold, such as:

- Limited understanding of the neurobiology of SUDs restricts the available potential targets for the same, raising the possibility that many of the probable target areas are being missed with the currently attainable pharmacotherapy.
- Lack of awareness, coupled with the stigma associated with mental illnesses leads to only a scanty number of needy patients reaching for treatment. The problem gets worse with the fact that of those reaching for help, adequate treatment is only given to a certain proportion.
- Lack of available services in terms of accessibility and cost-effectiveness, especially in congruence with the specific needs of each population, is another limiting factor.
- Due to the wide role of the psychosocial factors in SUD and the vast assortment of these factors from region to region leads to the narrowed reach of the available psychological measures to tackle them.

To tackle these issues, many novel treatment measures in terms of novel pharmacological agents, novel modes of their delivery, newer psychotherapeutic techniques and the use of technology are being studied worldwide to gather data on their efficacy, feasibility and cost-effectiveness.

TELEHEALTH

TH is the use of a technology-driven virtual platform to deliver the health-related interventions. TH is especially beneficial to populations such as those living in rural areas, those with mobility restrictions or small children.

TH is a broader term that includes *telemedicine* and *telerehabilitation*.

Telemedicine

It is defined as the practice of medicine via a remote electronic interface. Often, the term is used interchangeably with TH. There are several branches of telemedicine as per WHO: teledermatology, teleradiology, telepathology and telepsychology.

Telerehabilitation (TR)

TR is essentially a form of support to rehabilitation services using the various applications of telecommunication technology. Its origins can be dated back to time in 19th century when the number of physician visits were cut down with the use of telephone, as reported in the Lancet. Then, in 1910, came the description of a telestethoscope (Bashshur et al. 2009). In the past decade, there has been a significant upsurge in the evidence showing the role of telecommunication in the treatment of chronic diseases. This could be a very fertile area for use in mental illnesses as well, particularly the SUD (Dang et al. 2008; Wootton 2012)

Telerehabilitation Services

Parmanto and Saptono (2009) provide details of four types of TR services available as following:

Teleconsultation

Winters (2002) conceptualized teleconsultation as a 'face to face' tele-medicine model in which videoconferencing was used for interaction between a local provider and a client at one end and a rehabilitation expert at the other.

Telehomecare

Telehomecare can be understood as the delivery of service wherein the client is provided rehabilitation services at his home, coordinated by a clinician in liaisoning with various providers.

Telemonitoring

Telemonitoring is the application wherein the rehabilitation therapist sets up discreet monitoring for the client. However, some amount of interactivity between the client and the therapist is allowed by some of the telemonitoring approaches. Telemonitoring is one of the largest areas within TR which has the potential for expansion with the advent of wireless networks and also due to the availability of cost-effective and nonintrusive environmental sensors.

Teletherapy

In all likelihood, the most conspicuous application of TR services, teletherapy is the model of TR service delivery wherein therapeutic activities being managed by a therapist from a distance, are conducted in the home setting. The therapist mostly retains the ability to modify the therapy which can be done synchronously or asynchronously.

ASSESSMENT OF TECHNOLOGIES

While innovation and novelty lie at the foremost of TH and TR, it is concurrently essential to have guidelines for evaluation and monitoring of these technologies at the national and international level. Globally, there has been an edifying discussion on the need to develop a new framework for assessing TH technologies. Model for Assessment of Telemedicine Applications (MAST) was developed to provide a comprehensive assessment of TH technologies (Parmanto and Saptono 2009). The assessment process has three steps. First comes the preliminary feasibility assessment of the available technology. The second step involves assessment of the outcomes of the TH application in the domains of patient satisfaction, clinical effectiveness, safety, economic and socio-cultural aspects etc. Finally, in the third step, the transferability of the evidence to the local setting is considered. The MAST model is currently the most commonly used evaluation framework in European Union.

NOVEL APPLICATIONS AND INNOVATIONS IN SUD

Most of the recent literature for technological applications in the management of SUDs is restricted to its use in alcohol use disorder.

Alcohol Tracker Application

An application was devised for the purpose of self-management of alcohol consumption and later crowdsourcing was used to determine user perspectives (Zhang et al. 2016). The following contents were included while making the application:

- It enables individuals to note down and know the number of alcohol units they have consumed
- Immediate notification services, if users have exceeded the permissible limit for the day/or the week
- Calendar view of the total number of units of alcohol consumed on a weekly basis
- Immediate links with telephone service for consultation regarding alcohol issues for those who desire the same
- Basic information about alcohol abuse and dependence
- Knowledge about medical complications of substance abuse and dependence
- A feature on psychological therapies including functional analysis, behavioural goals' chart, etc.
- Integration of an AUDs Identification Test (AUDIT) questionnaire for self-monitoring and diagnosis.

The most useful functions perceived by users were notification services and information while psychotherapy was perceived to be least useful (Zhang et al. 2016).

Secure Continuous Remote Alcohol Monitor (SCRAMx)

Research on various aspects of AUDs has been limited by the scarcity of objective measures of drinking. The most common biochemical tests (breath, blood) are restricted to detecting drinking to just within several hours of consumption because alcohol is rapidly metabolized in the body. Consequently, self-report measures remain the only available means, which carry a high risk of bias. The introduction of transdermal alcohol detection technology to test alcohol drinking has addressed some of these limitations.

SCRAMx is an ankle bracelet having a transdermal electrochemical sensor that detects alcohol vapors near the skin. It has two circumvention detection sensors. A randomized controlled trial assessed the feasibility, acceptability, and adherence with this technology. Results showed good viability of the transdermal sensor among participants undergoing treatment for substance abuse. Eighty-one percent of participants reported that the bracelet helped them reduce drinking and 75 per cent further accepted that they would wear it for an extended duration, if required (Alessi, Barnett and Petry 2017).

Cognitive Behavioural Therapy (CBT)-Based Texting Intervention

Implementation of CBT in clinical settings is impeded by a lack of quality training and supervision. To overcome these issues, a 12-week CBT-based text messaging intervention (TXT-CBT) targeting antiretroviral (ART) compliance, risk behaviours and substance use in a population of HIV-infected substance users was devised by a group of researchers. A pilot randomized clinical trial on the same is underway. The intervention consists of a face-to-face counselling session based on CBT principles followed by daily messages for the next 12 weeks. The messages include medication reminders plus 2 or 3 additional messages on the topic of addiction recovery and associated risk behaviours. For drug relapse prevention 14 to 21 messages per week are dedicated to content pertaining to CBT skills, HIV risk behaviours and ART adherence.

Contingency Management for Alcohol Use Reduction Using a Transdermal Alcohol Sensor

Daily contingent reinforcement (CR) was compared with non-contingent reinforcement (NR) by a pilot randomized control design in which a transdermal alcohol sensor was used to detect alcohol use. Compared to NR (31.2%), CR had a higher proportion of days with no drinking detected (54.3%) during the intervention period. Four times more participants in CR drank below NIH low-risk drinking guidelines during intervention than did participants in NR. Conclusions from this study were that linking cash incentives to reduced drinking detected using a transdermal alcohol sensor can reduce heavy alcohol consumption (Barnett et al. 2017).

A Smarter Pathway for Delivering Cue Exposure Therapy (CET)

A CET and urge surfing coping skills (USCS)-based smartphone app has been developed by a group of researchers in Denmark. It contains an introduction, sessions with USCS, alcohol exposure videos for applying USCS and a results component providing an overview of the progress. Only on completion of one session is it possible for patients to proceed to the next session. The app keeps the Exposure icon locked until all other strategies have been completed.

A SYSTEMATIC REVIEW OF SMARTPHONE APPS

A systemic review was performed that evaluated smartphone apps to decrease alcohol consumption or treat AUD. Six apps were identified.

- Two of these apps, A-CHESS and LBMI-A showcased self-reported reductions in alcohol use
- Promillekoll and PartyPlanner failed to promote self-reported reductions in alcohol use, and
- HealthCall-S and Chimpshop require further evidence to reach a substantial conclusion on its efficacy.

Although advances in smartphone technology hold promise for developing interventions among individuals with AUD, further scientific evaluations are required to reach a conclusion on their clinical utility. Comprehensive data and conclusive evidence regarding the role of TR for mental illnesses are at best, scanty. Therefore, this area provides an exciting and unmissable window of opportunity to explore. Looking at the various aspects of management of SUD, the role of TR is mainly restricted to the long-term maintenance part, which is also the most challenging and neglected part.

EVIDENCE-BASED STUDIES OF SUBSTANCE USE DISORDERS

In the era of evidence-based medicine, it goes without saying that any new field aiming to make a mark shall need to be based on good research and evidence base. Along the same lines, with regards to TR in SUD, a range of research might turn to be useful. It has been shown that technology plays a great role in today's world in the acquisition of information leading to the formation of congruent habits. Technology might have its own risks like leading to an increase in illicit drug use, inculcation of addictive behaviours, facilitating the interaction of drug users etc. Therefore, it is essential that technology is appropriately developed and complemented with stringent monitoring and modification of the same, as and when required. Programmes such as 'CLIMATE' and 'Refuse to use' have shown great promise in preventing the young population from being addicted to various substances. Marsch and Borodovsky (2016) conducted a meta-analysis to compare technology-based interactions to face-to-face interactions which shows no difference between the efficiency of the two approaches (Barak et al. 2008). However, it is prudent at this point to emphasize that technological interventions are in no way meant to replace face-to-face therapeutic approach but to serve as an add-on and enrichment measure. Direct interaction with the therapist shall still be the primary and gold standard approach for management of SUD. The addition of technology-based interventions should be seen as a new dimension to the therapeutic repertoire. Though there has been the advent of TH modes of treatment for SUD in India in the form of video-conferencing psychotherapy sessions, online support groups etc., there still remains significant dearth of studies in the same from our country. These lacunae need to be filled upon with researches in various areas. Firstly, studies to test the efficacy and feasibility of the novel interventions in comparison to those already in place will be required. Secondly, qualitative research to gain insight into patient perceptions, requirements and experiences shall provide a foray into the user needs that need to be kept in mind while developing or revising technologies. Thirdly, virtually all the data on TH and TR currently comes from their application in chronic medical disorders. Therefore, it is high time for research base on same to grow in the field of mental health.

CHALLENGES AND ISSUES

Though the prospect of TR brings along an interesting and utilizable array of applications, there remain a set of challenges which must be addressed for smooth and efficient use of the TR in SUD. A recent report from Transatlantic Telehealth Research Network on personalized TH comprehensively presented the following challenges of TH services that can also be implicated in the area of SUD.

PERSONALIZATION OF HEALTH CARE

Individual SUD differs widely in terms of their genesis, epidemiology as per specific population; socio-demographic, clinical and psychosocial profile; co-morbid mental and medical disorders; and lastly their management approaches and needs. Any novel technology will need to take care of this wide spectrum. The technology will additionally need to have relevance to the particular individual and the family in order to ensure treatment adherence. Also, TR will need to take care to cater to the specific needs and desires of the patient. For instance, some patients might just want to use it a means of daily reminders to prevent lapses and would not prefer higher levels of intrusion into their life. On the other hand, some patients would want a more intensive intervention to help them through the daily obstacles in maintaining abstinence.

Similarly, there would be a set of patients who would want to use TH as an add-on means to their face-to-face visits to the mental health professionals. Also, the targets and expectations of different patients from the treatment process might vary. While some would prefer complete abstinence, some would want to limit to harm reduction, especially in AUDs. SUDs come with a huge variety of high-risk situations which predispose patients to make apparently irrelevant decisions and then leading to lapse and relapse. Complicating matters will be the presence of co-morbid mental and medical disorders which shall make the use highly subjective. The technology in concern will need to cater to the specific situations and solutions for the patient using it. Ease of use and access, aesthetics, the familiarity of technology will also be important factors to consider and a menu of options might be needed to tackle the same. So, a fine balance will be needed between the applications of the technology, illness and the patient profile and needs.

MATCHING PATIENTS WITH APPROPRIATE TECHNOLOGY

One of the biggest challenges of TH and TR shall be that they will need to cater to a population varying greatly in terms of age, education, cultural background, technological familiarity, cognitive and psychological mindedness. While the young and middle-aged population is more likely to be 'tech-savvy', the elderly are more likely to need easy to use technology for appropriate and adequate use.

The technology in concern will need to empower independence of the user to facilitate regular use. Another factor which needs to be addressed is that individual SUD coupled with the individual profile might demand differing technologies. For instance, alcoholics who consume alcohol in varying patterns and at various settings might require a different intervention compared to a tobacco user with a high frequency of consumption in a relatively same setting every day.

Similarly, recreational use with peers compared with use as a daily habit in solitude or company of family or use in varying socio-cultural milieus and norms might require differing technological features.

Therefore, technologies shall require great flexibility to able to reach out to the wide array of the population of users.

OPTIMAL AND SECURE USE OF HEALTH CARE DATA

While telecommunication technologies provide a broad opportunity of intervention and outreach, there shall remain concern regarding the optimal amount of personal data to be collected, privacy of the data collected and more importantly, the extent of involvement of third party carriers in data access. Third-party carriers will be necessary to ensure optimal use of the technology in concern, but at the same time, the data to be accessible to them and the associated indemnity will be an important issue to be addressed. The optimal and secure use of personal data will have high legal implications and hence, policymakers will have to ensure to take care of this aspect.

CREATING NEWER EDUCATION PARADIGMS

E-tools such as mobiles and handheld devices, along with large screens and desktops can be used as a means of education of patients regarding common and specific aspects of various SUD. However, the amount and level of information to be provided shall be an important area of concern.

In the modern era, when patients are likely to misinterpret available information on various diseases, it shall be imperative that such tools provide content which is helpful in patient gaining emotional and intellectual insight into their illness rather than instilling fear and lowering their confidence. Also, there exists a digital divide between patients which shall need to be taken care of by these technologies.

Smartphones and devices like the iPads are powerful and useful tools for professional education in the healthcare setting. Educational literature can be used with the help of smartphone technology to practice the evidence-based techniques that can also build a network amongst the professionals to interchange the information. However, it requires the collaborative approach of technology experts and health care providers.

COST-EFFECTIVENESS AND FEASIBILITY

Lastly, the technology in concern will need to be cost-effective to have a wide reach, especially more so because it is likely to target more, the rural population belonging to the lower socio-economic strata. Also, assessment of the feasibility of the individual technology at the target area and population will need to be ensured.

WAY FORWARD

Though TR brings with it loads of question marks, if taken care of in the right manner, they might well bring the much-needed boost in management of SUDs. Here, we discuss a list of possible solutions for the challenges and recommendations:

Multi-Sectoral Collaboration

As already mentioned, app developers shall be limited in their knowledge of evidence-based practices and patient profiles of SUDs. Therefore, a partnership with the experts in this field in all phases of technology development to assessment, regular use, monitoring and modifications shall be warranted. Also, collaboration with the policy and lawmakers will strengthen and shield this area of development and provide the right impetus to move ahead. Lastly, public health experts with their knowledge of ground-level issues of the target population can provide invaluable input into developing features which shall cater to the nuances of the various users. So, the collaboration between app developers or TH experts, experts in the field of SUD management i.e. mental health professionals, policy and lawmakers and experts from public health can go a long way in providing the right path to the development of TR.

Developing Guidelines and Sustainable Models

To obtain uniformity and encourage widespread use, formulating guidelines for technology makers as well as users, can go a long way in facilitation. Guidelines can provide a basic framework for manufacturers to keep in mind while developing newer technologies. It is also imperative the guidelines strike a fine balance between patient needs, legal and privacy concerns and creative freedom to app developers/ TH providers. Concurrently, to maintain cost-effectiveness, safety and long-term care, it shall be essential to develop sustainable models of TR. TH solutions need to incorporate multiple chronic disease paradigm as nowadays comorbid illnesses are more prevalent (Dinesen et al. 2016).

DISCUSSION

SUDs pose a significantly different widespread challenge compared to other mental disorders and medical disorders in general (Moulahoum et al. 2019). Right from their genesis to development and beyond, SUDs differ distinctively and encompass threat and trouble to all the stakeholders such as patients, clinicians, families and communities. The level of awareness among patients with SUD about the depth of the issue is staggeringly low. At the same time, the preventive approaches are also becoming more expensive due to the widening availability of different treatment measures (Michie and Abraham 2004). More so, even with the available avenues, full-scale implementation of preventive and therapeutic measures is hardly a reality due to the mismatch between demand and supply of human and financial resources along with the need for speciality training.

It goes unsaid that technology has reached an indispensable place in today's society. However, the enthusiasm of the wide applications of technology is balanced by its downsides. That being said, the wide availability of mobiles, Internet and other tools can be used to advantage at various levels for management of SUD including screening and assessment, delivering interventions, monitoring and promoting awareness (Marsch 2012).

Furthermore, technology-driven interventions provide privacy, easy accessibility, convenience to use that further enhances the acceptance of problems and motivation to change (Copeland 2011; Moulahoum et al. 2019). However, there remain concerns such as ethical issues, matching appropriate technology with the user, flexibility and personalizing health care which needs to be kept in mind while contemplating and implementing technology for the management of SUD. There is a growing need for exploratory and confirmatory research in the arena of technology-based management of SUDs. Future researches in different areas (feasibility, comparative and qualitative studies) shall reap great information and insights into this newly emerging field.

CONCLUSION

TR provides a very exciting and much needed added-dimension for tackling the gigantic issue of SUDs. However, the same shall need to carefully develop and extensively researched upon to develop a good literature base to enter into the foray of evidence-based medicine. Given the magnitude of the problem and the marked shortcomings of currently available measures in meeting the demands, TR might provide the much-needed silver lining.

REFERENCES

Alessi, Sheila M., Nancy P. Barnett, and Nancy M. Petry. 2017. 'Experiences with SCRAMx Alcohol Monitoring Technology in 100 Alcohol Treatment Outpatients.' *Drug and Alcohol Dependence* 178 (September): 417–424. doi: 10.1016/j.drugalcdep.2017.05.031

American Psychiatric Association. n.d. *Diagnostic and Statistical Manual of Mental Disorders (DSM–5®)* (Google Books). Available at: https://books.google.co.in/books?hl=en&lr=&id=-JivBAAAQBAJ&oi=fnd&pg=PT18&dq=DSM 5&ots = ceTT70PGya&sig = JY9uH0M3Q1wg4MAXbe5kcSP8qc4&redir_esc = y#v = onepage&q = DSM–5&f = false (accessed on 30 September 2019).

Barak, Azy, Liat Hen, Meyran Boniel-Nissim, and Na'ama Shapira. 2008. 'A Comprehensive Review and a Meta-Analysis of the Effectiveness of Internet-Based Psychotherapeutic Interventions.' *Journal of Technology in Human Services* 26 (2–4): 109–160. doi: 10.1080/15228830802094429

Barnett, Nancy P., Mark A. Celio, Jennifer W. Tidey, James G. Murphy, Suzanne M. Colby, and Robert M. Swift. 2017. 'A Preliminary Randomized Controlled Trial of Contingency Management for Alcohol Use Reduction Using a Transdermal Alcohol Sensor: Contingency Management for Alcohol Use Reduction.' *Addiction* 112 (6): 1025–1035. doi: 10.1111/add.13767

Bashshur, Rashid L., Gary W. Shannon, Elizabeth A. Krupinski, Jim Grigsby, Joseph C. Kvedar, Ronald S. Weinstein, Jay H. Sanders, et al. 2009. 'National Telemedicine Initiatives: Essential to Healthcare Reform.' *Telemedicine and E-Health* 15 (6): 600–610. doi: 10.1089/tmj.2009.9960

Copeland, Jan. 2011. 'Application of Technology in the Prevention and Treatment of Substance Use Disorders and Related Problems: Opportunities and Challenges.' *Substance Use & Misuse* 46 (1): 112–113. doi: 10.3109/10826084.2011.521423

Dang, Stuti, Nilber Remon, Julia Harris, Julie Malphurs, Lauran Sandals, Angeles Lozada Cabrera, and Nicole Nedd. 2008. 'Care Coordination Assisted by Technology for Multiethnic Caregivers of Persons with Dementia: A Pilot Clinical Demonstration Project on Caregiver Burden and Depression.' *Journal of Telemedicine and Telecare* 14 (8): 443–447. doi: 10.1258/jtt.2008.080608

Dinesen, Birthe, Brandie Nonnecke, David Lindeman, Egon Toft, Kristian Kidholm, Kamal Jethwani, Heather M. Young, et al. 2016. 'Personalized Telehealth in the Future: A Global Research Agenda.' *Journal of Medical Internet Research* 18 (3): e53. doi: 10.2196/jmir.5257

Marsch, Lisa A. 2012. 'Leveraging Technology to Enhance Addiction Treatment and Recovery.' *Journal of Addictive Diseases* 31 (3): 313–318. doi: 10.1080/10550887.2012.694606

Marsch, Lisa A., and Jacob T. Borodovsky. 2016. 'Technology-Based Interventions for Preventing and Treating Substance Use Among Youth.' *Child and Adolescent Psychiatric Clinics of North America* 25 (4): 755–768. doi: 10.1016/j.chc.2016.06.005

Mbuba, Caroline K., Anthony K. Ngugi, Charles R. Newton, and Julie A. Carter. 2008. 'The Epilepsy Treatment Gap in Developing Countries: A Systematic Review of the Magnitude, Causes and Intervention Strategies.' *Epilepsia* 49 (9): 1491–1503. doi: 10.1111/j.1528-1167.2008.01693

Michie, Susan, and Charles Abraham. 2004. 'Interventions to Change Health Behaviours: Evidence-Based or Evidence-Inspired?' *Psychology & Health* 19 (1): 29–49. doi: 10.1080/0887044031000141199

Moulahoum, Hichem, Figen Zihnioglu, Suna Timur, and Hakan Coskunol. 2019. 'Novel Technologies in Detection, Treatment and Prevention of Substance Use Disorders.' *Journal of Food and Drug Analysis* 27 (1): 22–31. doi: 10.1016/j.jfda.2018.09.003

Murthy, R. Srinivasa. 2017. 'National Mental Health Survey of India 2015–2016.' *Indian Journal of Psychiatry* 59 (1): 21. doi: 10.4103/psychiatry.IndianJPsychiatry_102_17

Parmanto, Bambang, and Andi Saptono. 2009. 'Telerehabilitation: State-of-the-Art from an Informatics Perspective.' *International Journal of Telerehabilitation* 1 (1): 73–84.

Winters, Jack M. 2002. 'Telerehabilitation Research: Emerging Opportunities.' *Annual Review of Biomedical Engineering* 4 (1): 287–320. doi: 10.1146/annurev.bioeng.4.112801.121923

Wootton, Richard. 2012. 'Twenty Years of Telemedicine in Chronic Disease Management—an Evidence Synthesis.' *Journal of Telemedicine and Telecare* 18 (4): 211–220. doi: 10.1258/jtt.2012.120219

Zhang, Melvyn W. B., John Ward, John J. B. Ying, Fang Pan, and Roger C. M. Ho. 2016. 'The Alcohol Tracker Application: An Initial Evaluation of User Preferences.' *BMJ Innovations* 2 (1): 8–13. doi: 10.1136/bmjinnov-2015-000087

ABOUT THE EDITOR AND CONTRIBUTORS

EDITOR

Sanjeev Kumar Gupta, PhD, is Clinical Psychologist at the All India Institute of Speech and Hearing, Mysuru, India. His clinical and research work includes child and adolescent mental health, cognitive behaviour therapy, mindfulness meditation and telerehabilitation for service delivery in Clinical Psychology. His books include Emerging Trends in the Diagnosis and Intervention of Neurodevelopmental Disorders and Handbook of Research on Psychosocial Perspectives of Human Communication Disorder. He has completed one research project, contributed five chapters and published 15 articles in refereed journals. He has chaired scientific sessions and presented many research papers both at national and international conferences. He has also conducted many workshops and training programmes for professionals and caregivers of children with neurodevelopmental disorders.

CONTRIBUTORS

Abdulaziz Saleh Almudhi works as an Assistant Professor in Medical Rehabilitation Sciences at King Khalid University (KKU), Saudi Arabia and as a Consultant of speech-language pathology within KKU Medical City. He obtained a BSc degree in speech pathology and audiology from King Saud University in 2006 and later received MSc in clinical communication disorders from Manchester Metropolitan University

the form of video-conferencing psychotherapy sessions, online support groups etc., there still remains significant dearth of studies in the same from our country. These lacunae need to be filled upon with researches in various areas. Firstly, studies to test the efficacy and feasibility of the novel interventions in comparison to those already in place will be required. Secondly, qualitative research to gain insight into patient perceptions, requirements and experiences shall provide a foray into the user needs that need to be kept in mind while developing or revising technologies. Thirdly, virtually all the data on TH and TR currently comes from their application in chronic medical disorders. Therefore, it is high time for research base on same to grow in the field of mental health.

CHALLENGES AND ISSUES

Though the prospect of TR brings along an interesting and utilizable array of applications, there remain a set of challenges which must be addressed for smooth and efficient use of the TR in SUD. A recent report from Transatlantic Telehealth Research Network on personalized TH comprehensively presented the following challenges of TH services that can also be implicated in the area of SUD.

PERSONALIZATION OF HEALTH CARE

Individual SUD differs widely in terms of their genesis, epidemiology as per specific population; socio-demographic, clinical and psychosocial profile; co-morbid mental and medical disorders; and lastly their management approaches and needs. Any novel technology will need to take care of this wide spectrum. The technology will additionally need to have relevance to the particular individual and the family in order to ensure treatment adherence. Also, TR will need to take care to cater to the specific needs and desires of the patient. For instance, some patients might just want to use it a means of daily reminders to prevent lapses and would not prefer higher levels of intrusion into their life. On the other hand, some patients would want a more intensive intervention to help them through the daily obstacles in maintaining abstinence.

Similarly, there would be a set of patients who would want to use TH as an add-on means to their face-to-face visits to the mental health professionals. Also, the targets and expectations of different patients from the treatment process might vary. While some would prefer complete abstinence, some would want to limit to harm reduction, especially in AUDs. SUDs come with a huge variety of high-risk situations which predispose patients to make apparently irrelevant decisions and then leading to lapse and relapse. Complicating matters will be the presence of co-morbid mental and medical disorders which shall make the use highly subjective. The technology in concern will need to cater to the specific situations and solutions for the patient using it. Ease of use and access, aesthetics, the familiarity of technology will also be important factors to consider and a menu of options might be needed to tackle the same. So, a fine balance will be needed between the applications of the technology, illness and the patient profile and needs.

MATCHING PATIENTS WITH APPROPRIATE TECHNOLOGY

One of the biggest challenges of TH and TR shall be that they will need to cater to a population varying greatly in terms of age, education, cultural background, technological familiarity, cognitive and psychological mindedness. While the young and middle-aged population is more likely to be 'tech-savvy', the elderly are more likely to need easy to use technology for appropriate and adequate use.

The technology in concern will need to empower independence of the user to facilitate regular use. Another factor which needs to be addressed is that individual SUD coupled with the individual profile might demand differing technologies. For instance, alcoholics who consume alcohol in varying patterns and at various settings might require a different intervention compared to a tobacco user with a high frequency of consumption in a relatively same setting every day.

Similarly, recreational use with peers compared with use as a daily habit in solitude or company of family or use in varying socio-cultural milieus and norms might require differing technological features.

Therefore, technologies shall require great flexibility to able to reach out to the wide array of the population of users.

OPTIMAL AND SECURE USE OF HEALTH CARE DATA

While telecommunication technologies provide a broad opportunity of intervention and outreach, there shall remain concern regarding the optimal amount of personal data to be collected, privacy of the data collected and more importantly, the extent of involvement of third party carriers in data access. Third-party carriers will be necessary to ensure optimal use of the technology in concern, but at the same time, the data to be accessible to them and the associated indemnity will be an important issue to be addressed. The optimal and secure use of personal data will have high legal implications and hence, policymakers will have to ensure to take care of this aspect.

CREATING NEWER EDUCATION PARADIGMS

E-tools such as mobiles and handheld devices, along with large screens and desktops can be used as a means of education of patients regarding common and specific aspects of various SUD. However, the amount and level of information to be provided shall be an important area of concern.

In the modern era, when patients are likely to misinterpret available information on various diseases, it shall be imperative that such tools provide content which is helpful in patient gaining emotional and intellectual insight into their illness rather than instilling fear and lowering their confidence. Also, there exists a digital divide between patients which shall need to be taken care of by these technologies.

Smartphones and devices like the iPads are powerful and useful tools for professional education in the healthcare setting. Educational literature can be used with the help of smartphone technology to practice the evidence-based techniques that can also build a network amongst the professionals to interchange the information. However, it requires the collaborative approach of technology experts and health care providers.

COST-EFFECTIVENESS AND FEASIBILITY

Lastly, the technology in concern will need to be cost-effective to have a wide reach, especially more so because it is likely to target more, the rural population belonging to the lower socio-economic strata. Also, assessment of the feasibility of the individual technology at the target area and population will need to be ensured.

WAY FORWARD

Though TR brings with it loads of question marks, if taken care of in the right manner, they might well bring the much-needed boost in management of SUDs. Here, we discuss a list of possible solutions for the challenges and recommendations:

Multi-Sectoral Collaboration

As already mentioned, app developers shall be limited in their knowledge of evidence-based practices and patient profiles of SUDs. Therefore, a partnership with the experts in this field in all phases of technology development to assessment, regular use, monitoring and modifications shall be warranted. Also, collaboration with the policy and lawmakers will strengthen and shield this area of development and provide the right impetus to move ahead. Lastly, public health experts with their knowledge of ground-level issues of the target population can provide invaluable input into developing features which shall cater to the nuances of the various users. So, the collaboration between app developers or TH experts, experts in the field of SUD management i.e. mental health professionals, policy and lawmakers and experts from public health can go a long way in providing the right path to the development of TR.

Developing Guidelines and Sustainable Models

To obtain uniformity and encourage widespread use, formulating guidelines for technology makers as well as users, can go a long way in facilitation. Guidelines can provide a basic framework for manufacturers to keep in mind while developing newer technologies. It is also imperative the guidelines strike a fine balance between patient needs,

in 2010 and a PhD in clinical language sciences from the University of Reading in 2014. He has more than 5 years of teaching experiences and has published several articles in international journals.

Abhishek B. P. works as Lecturer in speech sciences in the Department of Speech-Language Sciences at AIISH. He completed his Master's in Speech and Hearing in the year 2009 and received PhD in Speech-Language Pathology in 2015, both from the University of Mysore. He has around 7 years of teaching experience and has published several articles in national and international journals.

Rakesh C. V. is a Junior Research Fellow at the AIISH, Mysuru.

Husna Firdose is working as an Assistant Professor in Audiology, Department of Hearing Studies, Dr S. R. Chandrasekhar Institute of Speech and Hearing, Bengaluru.

Rachel C. Francis has a Master's degree in audiology and speech-language pathology. She is the recipient of Sri MPC Shetty Gold Medal for securing highest marks in MASLP course for the academic year 2012–2013. Since then, she has worked as a school-based speech-language pathologist, research associate and SLP-Grade-I for various research projects. Presently she is research officer at AIISH, Mysuru.

Pebbili Gopikishore currently works as Assistant Professor at AIISH, Mysuru. He did his PhD in speech-language pathology. He has more than 11 years of teaching and research experience in the field of speech pathology. He was assistant coordinator for the BASLP programme at NSCB Medical College, Jabalpur, for a couple of years. He has 17 publications and several presentations in national and international platforms to his credit. He has completed several projects and was a resource person at various conferences. He has received best presenter awards at various workshops and seminars. He is currently working in the area of voice disorders.

S. P. Goswami holds PhD in speech and hearing and also holds PGDHRM and MBA in health care management. He is the first speech and hearing professional to receive the prestigious CV Raman fellowship from UGC, Government of India, as visiting scholar at College of Applied Health Sciences, Department of Speech & Hearing Science, the University of Illinois at Urbana-Champaign, USA. Presently, he works as Professor and Head, Telecenter for Persons with Communication Disorders, and formerly worked as Head Department of Speech-Language Pathology Academic coordinator, Clinical services, AIISH, Mysuru. He has more than 19 years of academic, clinical, research and administrative experience. He works in the areas of aphasia, ageing and neuro-cognitive communication disorders in adults and elderly. He has completed more than 22 research projects and is presently working on five projects funded by national and international bodies. He has published more than 35 research articles in national and international journals, 25 in-house publications and 19 books/chapters/tools/tests with ISBN numbers. Three candidates have been awarded PhD and eight are presently pursuing their doctorate programme under his guidance. He was instrumental in framing the document for the scope of practice in audiology and speech-language pathology in India in 2010. He has served at the national forum for capacity building, matters for framing policy, NAAC and other national bodies in the area of speech-language pathology and audiology. He has served ISHA for more than 12 years in the capacity of Honorary Editor, Secretary, Treasurer and Joint Secretary.

Pratiksha Gupta has been practicing as a private SLPA in India since 2007. She is the founder and director of 1SpecialPlace, India's leading organization in telepractice and cloud-based technologies. She is a PhD Fellow at UKZN, South Africa, did her MSc from UCL, London, and is the Gold Medalist (in BSc) from AIISH, India. She has developed various apps and a software for speech therapy created numerous resource materials in speech-language pathology and India's first training course in telepractice. In 2018, she and her team were awarded a special prize by Amazon for their artificial intelligence app called Speech Doctor.

Tanu Gupta is presently serving as a Clinical Psychologist at the Department of Psychiatry, All India Institute of Medical Sciences (AIIMS), Jodhpur. She earned MPhil in clinical psychology from the

Institute of Human Behaviour and Allied Sciences, Delhi, and obtained PhD in clinical psychology from AIIMS, New Delhi. She has been awarded doctoral fellowship from Indian Council of Social Science Research, New Delhi, and a senior research fellowship from Indian Council Medical Research, New Delhi. She has worked as a faculty with National Institute of Mentally Handicapped (NIMH), regional centre, New Delhi. She has supervised graduate and postgraduate psychology interns and mentored them for their thesis work as a guide. She has worked in collaboration with many international agencies such as the National Institute of Health (NIH), USA, and Brown University, USA. She has actively participated in various national and international conferences and workshops. She has written numbers of chapters in textbooks and has published articles in peer-reviewed journals. Her specific areas of interest are cognitive behaviour therapy, child and adolescent psychotherapy, and stress management.

Chandni Jain works as a Reader in the Department of Audiology at AIISH, Mysuru.

Saransh Jain works as a Lecturer in audiology at the JSS Institute of Speech and Hearing, Mysuru since last 7 years. He has secured gold medal from the University of Mysore for his postgraduation in speech and hearing, from the University of Rajasthan for postgraduation in clinical psychology and for undergraduation in speech and hearing. He has also received outstanding clinician award from READS society for hearing impaired children, Jaipur. His research interests include understanding the perception of speech in normal and differently abled individuals, psychoacoustic processing in the human auditory system, auditory processing disorders, cognitive processing abilities and its association with audition. His research experience includes two book chapters in research handbooks, 17 international paper publications in peer-reviewed journals, 5 national paper publications and 32 paper presentations in national and international conferences. He had also guided 16 master's level dissertation students and presently guiding 4 more students for the academic year 2017–2018. He is also pursuing his PhD in understanding the temporal processing abilities by hearing-impaired individuals.

Megha K. N. is a Research Officer at the Department of Audiology, AIISH, Mysuru.

Vimala Jayakrishna Kasturi works as Assistant Professor at Naseema Institute of Speech and Hearing, Bengaluru, is a postgraduate in speech-language pathology from AIISH. She has worked as a research officer at AIISH. Her research was focused on developing an app-based cognitive-linguistic rehabilitation for persons with aphasia in Indian languages in collaboration with The Learning Corp, which is a leading firm working towards building the next generation in digital thera-peutics. She has published and presented her researches at various national and international platforms. She has also served as resource person for a few national conferences in India.

G. Malar has done dual graduation in rehabilitation sciences (BRSc) and special education (BEdSplEd-HI), post-graduation in reha-bilitation sciences (MRSc specializing in hearing impairment) from Bharathidasan University, Tamil Nadu, and a doctorate in speech pathology and audiology (following experimental study on dys-praxia among children with hearing impairment) from NIMHANS, Bengaluru, as a JRF. Currently, she is working as Reader in Special Education at AIISH, Mysuru, for the past 16 years. She, along with eight years of experience in active research and eighteen years of teaching as a master trainer, has over two decades of work experience.

Santosh Maruthy is an Associate Professor and Head of the Department of Speech-Language Sciences at AIISH, Mysuru. He has completed his postdoctoral research from the Department of Speech and Hearing Sciences, University of Washington, USA. His areas of interests are fluency disorders, voice disorders, speech and language processing.

Vijaya Kumar Narne is currently pursuing his Post-Doc at the Department of Clinical Research, South Denmark University, Denmark. He has secured his postgraduation and PhD in audiology from the University of Mysore. His research interests include under-standing the perception of speech in normal and differently able individuals, psychoacoustic and electrophysiology in the human auditory system. He has secured 8 grants from AIISH and one extramural grant from Cognitive Science Initiative, Department of Science and Technology. Further, he collaborates nationally and internationally with eminent professors in the field of audiology. To his credit, he has 24 publications in highly ranked international peer-reviewed journals. He had also guided 20 Master's level dissertations.

Attuluri Navya completed PhD in speech-language pathology from AIISH and currently works as a Research Officer. She was a teaching faculty for a couple of years and presented research papers and chaired scientific sessions at various national and international conferences. She has received the best paper presenter award and international travel grants. She has also published 21 scientific articles and acts as a reviewer for several national and international journals. She was a member of BOS at Madhya Pradesh Medical Science University (MPMSU). She dealt with patients with various speech and language disorders especially in the area of cleft lip and palate and swallowing disorders.

Prashanth Prabhu P. received his Master's in audiology from the University of Mysore. He is currently working as Assistant Professor in audiology at AIISH, Mysuru. His major interest is in auditory neuropathy spectrum disorder (ANSD). He has published several research articles and has had conference presentations in the area. He is currently working on developing hearing aid modification strategies to help individuals with ANSD.

Yashaswini R. has completed MSc in speech-language pathology from AIISH. She has also submitted her doctorate thesis in speech-language pathology to the University of Mysore. Currently, she works as Clinical Supervisor, TCPD at AIISH.

Hemanth N. Shetty completed his doctoral program from AIISH, Mysuru. He has been working as a Reader in Audiology at AIISH. Published his articles on amplification and rehabilitation in high impact factor journals. His research findings have been disseminated in various conferences. He has delivered a talk as a resource person on workshops and seminars. He has developed many software programs, to name a few (a) audiology client database management system (CDMS) for the Department of Audiology, (b) teaching and training simulator for audiological evaluation, (c) tinnitus software which includes evaluation and the contemporary treatment strategy 'frequency discrimination task in a game format' to encourage the patient to use it consistently and improves intrinsic motivation, and (d) cognitive software includes modules on listening effort and semantic information processing (SIP). Currently, he is working on developing computerized audiometer. This will be utilized to conduct the audiological evaluation in individuals who resides in the underserved community.

Kartik Singhai is currently pursuing his residency from the Department of Psychiatry, AIIMS, Jodhpur, after having passed his graduation from B. J. Government Medical College, Pune. His interest areas include mood and anxiety disorders, de-addiction psychiatry, mental well-being of college students, cognitive behaviour therapy and qualitative research. He is a part of multiple ongoing research projects in the field of mood disorders and has a number of publications in national and international journals to his credit. He has been actively participating in various conferences, workshops and symposiums. Furthermore, he is a blog writer at 'The Abhivyakti Columns-Perspectives' (AIIMS Jodhpur Literature Club).

G. Swetha has completed her Master's in speech-language pathology and audiology from Mysore University and MSc in psychology from Madras University. She has a wide variety of experience in dealing with children and adults with varied communication disorders since 2008. She was actively involved in research activities and guided around 13 publications, various scientific papers at national level conferences which have also won various awards. She has guided several journal clubs and dissertations of the postgraduate programme and also served as a resource person at various national level conferences. Currently, she is working as a senior language pathologist at Billabong High International School, Noida.

INDEX